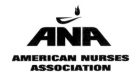

AMERICAN NURSES
ASSOCIATION

MW01077804

Scope AND
Standards
OF PRACTICE

Cardiovascular
Nursing

2ND EDITION

American Nurses Association
Silver Spring, Maryland
2015

The American Nurses Association (ANA) is a national professional association. This publication, *Cardiovascular Nursing: Scope and Standards of Practice, Second Edition*, reflects the thinking of the practice specialty of cardiovascular nursing on various issues and should be reviewed in conjunction with state board of nursing policies and practices. State law, rules, and regulations govern the practice of nursing, while *Cardiovascular Nursing: Scope and Standards of Practice, Second Edition*, guides cardiovascular nurses in the application of their professional skills and responsibilities.

The American Nurses Association is the only full-service professional organization representing the interests of the nation's 3.1 million registered nurses through its constituent/state nurses associations and its organizational affiliates. The ANA advances the nursing profession by fostering high standards of nursing practice, promoting the rights of nurses in the workplace, projecting a positive and realistic view of nursing, and by lobbying the Congress and regulatory agencies on health care issues affecting nurses and the public.

American Nurses Association
8515 Georgia Avenue, Suite 400
Silver Spring, MD 20910-3492
1-800-274-4ANA
www.NursingWorld.org

Published by Nursesbooks.org
The Publishing Program of ANA
www.Nursesbooks.org/

Library of Congress Cataloging-in-Publication Data on file with the Library of Congress.

ISBN-13: 978-1-55810-623-9   SAN: 851-3481   1.5K   06/2015

First printing: June 2015

Contents

Contributors

Workgroup Members

Eileen Handberg, PhD, ARNP-BC, FAHA, FACC – Chairperson
American College of Cardiology representative

Cynthia Arslanian-Engoren, PhD, RN, ACNS-BC, FAHA, FAAN
American Heart Association Council on Cardiovascular and Stroke
    Nursing representative

Linda Baas, PhD, RN, ACNP, CHFN, FAHA
American Association of Heart Failure Nurses representative

Cheryl Dennison Himmelfarb, PhD, RN, ANP, FAHA, FPCNA, FAAN
Preventive Cardiovascular Nurses Association representative

Melanie T. Gura, MSN, RN, CNS, CCDS, FHRS, FAHA, AACC
Heart Rhythm Society representative

Deborah Klein, MSN, RN, ACNS-BC, CCRN, CHFN, FAHA
American Association of Critical-Care Nurses representative

Wilhemina Maslanek, MSN, RN, ACNP-BC
International Transplant Nurses Society

Caryl Mayo, MS, RN, FNGNA
National Gerontological Nursing Association representative

Maria R. Molina, MSN, ACNP-BC, AGACNP-BC, CCRN
International Transplant Nurses Society

Mary Rummell, MN, RN, CPNP, CNS, FAHA
Society of Pediatric Cardiovascular Nurses representative

Julie Stanik-Hutt, PhD, ACNP, GNP, CCNS, FAANP, FAAN
American Association of Nurse Practitioners representative

Kathleen K. Zarling, MS, APRN, ACNS-BC, MAACVPR, FPCNA
American Association of Cardiovascular and Pulmonary Rehabilitation
    representative

ANA Staff

Carol J. Bickford, PhD, RN-BC, CPHIMS, FAAN, Content editor

Eric Wurzbacher, BA, Project editor

Maureen Cones, Esq., Legal counsel

Yvonne Humes, MSA, Project coordinator

Contributing Organizations

Representatives of the following groups comprised the workgroup. These groups also have endorsed this publication. The mission statements and other information about each group are available at the URLs below each logo.

AMERICAN
ASSOCIATION
of CRITICAL-CARE
NURSES

http://www.aacn.org/

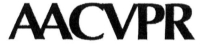

American Association of Cadiovascular
and Pulmonary Rehabilitation

Promoting Health & Preventing Disease

https://www.aacvpr.org/

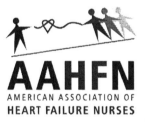

AMERICAN ASSOCIATION OF
HEART FAILURE NURSES

https://www.aahfn.org/

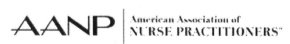

http://www.aanp.org/

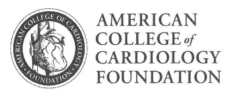

http://www.acc.org/

AHA Council on Cardiovascular Nursing and Stroke Nursing

http://my.americanheart
.org/professional/Councils/
Councils_UCM_316892_
SubHomePage.jsp

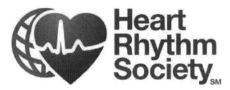

http://www.hrsonline.org/

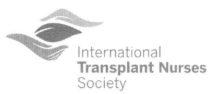

http://www.itns.org/

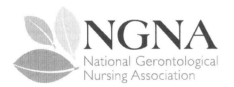

http://www.ngna.org/

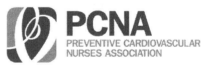

http://pcna.net/

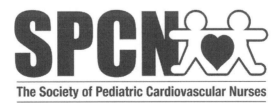

http://spcnonline.com/

Introduction

Cardiovascular disease remains the *primary* cause of death and disability in both men and women worldwide. According to the 2015 American Heart Association (AHA) statistical update on heart disease and stroke, cardiovascular disease is responsible for more than 31.9% of all deaths annually in America and claims more lives than cancer and pneumonia/respiratory disease combined (AHA, 2015, e129). Nearly 84 million adults, including men and women of all races, in the United States are currently living with some form of cardiovascular disease. The AHA projects that by 2030, 43.9% of the U.S. population will have some form of cardiovascular disease. An estimated 42.2 million of these persons will be 60 years old or older. These numbers are decreasing, however, and by some estimates could be reduced by another 44.47% with increased use of evidence-based medical and nursing interventions targeted at secondary prevention and management of risk impacted by lifestyle and environmental factors (AHA, 2015, e129).

Congenital heart disease, the most common type of birth defect, accounts for more than one-third of all birth defects and occurs in nearly 1% of births (about 40,000) in the United States each year. As the most common cause of infant mortality, congenital heart disease accounts for 23.8% of deaths in infants with birth defects and is responsible for more than half of the $2.4 billion spent annually on care for birth defects. The most expensive neonatal hospital charges (nearly $200,000) are for congenital heart defects (Centers for Disease Control and Prevention [CDC], n.d.).

With improved surgical outcomes and medical management of infants and children with congenital heart disease, adults with congenital heart disease now outnumber children with this problem. The prevalence of adults living with congenital heart disease is 1 in 150. The death rate from congenital heart defects has declined 21.39% over the previous 30 years, with deaths occurring at progressively older ages (CDC, n.d.).

Diseases of the cardiovascular system are responsible for much of the economic burden of health care in the United States and other developed countries. The estimated medical and disability cost for treatment of cardiovascular diseases in 2011 was $320.1 billion. By 2030, an estimated 44% of the U.S. population will have some form of cardiovascular disease, and the total direct medical costs will increase from $396 billion to $918 billion. The indirect costs attributable to lost productivity are estimated to reach $290 billion in 2030, an increase of 58% (AHA, 2015).

The prevalence and management of cardiovascular health and risk factors are major health and economic burdens in the United States. The findings of the Framingham study helped define the understanding of cardiovascular risk and began the scientific journey to develop effective treatment strategies. Over time, the focus has increasingly been directed toward individuals and populations to promote lifestyle changes. Attention is also directed at the familial and genetic basis of cardiovascular disease, as data suggest that most cardiovascular risk factors have at least moderate heritability. Targeted areas of study include the development of genomic risk scores, with genetic counseling aimed at the identification and management of cardiovascular disease (AHA, 2015; Musunuru et al., 2015).

Identification of cardiovascular risk factors and hyperlipidemia management starts in childhood, as prevention and management differ between children and adults. Although cholesterol screening in adolescents is particularly challenging, and high cholesterol is not the only risk factor for cardiovascular disease, lipid profiles should be obtained once when a person is between 9 and 11 years and again between 17 and 20 years of age. Selected screening is recommended for children 2 years of age and older who have a family history of early cardiovascular disease and hypercholesterolemia (Kavey, Simmons-Morton, & deJesus, 2011).

Over the past 70 years, nurses have been integral members of care teams for patients with cardiovascular health needs in a wide variety of healthcare environments. Heart surgery began in 1944 with the first palliative procedure for "blue" babies. The first open-heart surgery was performed in 1955 to repair a congenital defect. Nurses in the 1950s helped develop specialized operating rooms for heart and lung surgery and cardiac catheterization laboratories. In 1957, one of the world's first coronary care units (CCUs) opened in America. At that time the units were called "heart rooms" or constant care units because nurses provided care around the clock for these vulnerable patients. Both surgical and post-myocardial infarction patients were treated in this environment. Coronary care units provided a model for specialized care where nurses learned about arrhythmia recognition and early defibrillation. Infants and children were typically isolated in specialized areas of pediatric wards, whose nursing staff acquired high levels of skill in yet another important area of cardiovascular health care. As the science of cardiovascular nursing emerged, expectations of care rose among the public, patients, and the healthcare professions.

Today the field of cardiovascular nursing is rich with opportunities for registered nurses and advanced practice registered nurses to affect the lives of patients and families. Nursing practice encompasses the vast needs of patients across the life span, from newborns and children to the elderly. The genetic influences on cardiac disease are gaining increased attention; similarly, obesity prevention starts in infancy and carries on throughout the life span. Encouraging the community to be physically active, eat healthfully, and stop smoking can significantly reduce the morbidity and mortality associated with cardiovascular disease and places registered nurses and advanced practice nurses at the front lines to help the public achieve the goals of Healthy People 2020 (https://www.HealthyPeople.gov). Cardiovascular nurses lead the development, coordination, and management of many of these prevention efforts.

The increasing global burden of cardiovascular disease, an expanding ethnically diverse population, and an aging population with multiple comorbidities characterize today's healthcare environment. These changes, combined with limited healthcare resources and workforce shortages of physicians and nurses, provide an abundance of challenges and opportunities for cardiovascular nurses to provide leadership in the prevention and management of cardiovascular disease. Given the limited number of providers to care for this expanding population, utilization of all members of a collaborative team practicing to the full scope of their education and licensure is vital to the health and well-being of all cardiovascular patients. Excellence in cardiovascular nursing requires advanced cardiovascular knowledge and skills, including knowledge of cardiovascular gender differences. This document describes the knowledge base, scope of practice, and standards of practice and professional performance, and provides a framework for developing cardiovascular nursing educational curricula.

Scope of Practice of Cardiovascular Nursing

Definition of Cardiovascular Nursing

Cardiovascular nursing is specialized nursing care focused on the optimization of cardiovascular health across the life span and in diverse practice settings. Cardiovascular nursing care includes education, prevention, detection, and treatment of cardiovascular disease in individuals, families, communities, and populations.

Cardiovascular nurses are registered nurses who focus on health promotion, genetic risk assessment, disease and injury prevention, sign and symptom recognition, cardiovascular disease management, and self-care knowledge and adherence to improve patient outcomes for those at risk or living with cardiovascular disease and illness. Cardiovascular nurses provide evidence-based practice to improve patient functional capacity and quality of life, and to enhance the heart-health of communities. Cardiovascular nurses develop, implement, and participate in nursing and interprofessional cardiovascular research to address the knowledge gaps in the prevention, diagnosis, and treatment of cardiovascular disease. Practice-based research by cardiovascular nurses provides a better understanding of the impact of healthcare practices and nursing interventions on patient outcomes.

Many titles or terms describe patients across organizations and settings, including *healthcare consumers, clients, individuals, families, caregivers, groups, communities*, and *populations*. For this professional resource, *patient* serves as the preferred term and includes, depending on the context of use, individuals, families, groups, communities, and/or populations.

Key elements of cardiovascular nursing include:

■ Development of programs that promote heart health;

■ Education and counseling about heart health;

■ Interventions that reduce risk factors;

■ Individualized, evidence-based interventions that maintain or improve physiologic, psychological, and psychosocial health;

■ Interventions that facilitate and optimize behavioral change and treatment adherence over time;

■ Conduct of research; and

■ Advocacy to support patients and families during the planning, implementation, and evaluation of their care.

The high incidence and prevalence of cardiovascular disease, the obesity epidemic, the dramatic growth in the population of older adults and adults with congenital heart disease, and the increasing costs associated with advanced treatment technologies are all contributing to escalating healthcare costs. Cardiovascular nurses play a key role in providing, coordinating, and improving cost-effective quality patient care across all sites where cardiovascular care is provided.

Cardiovascular care at the healthcare organization delivery level emphasizes collaborative practices, disease management, education, research, and administration to ensure quality care. Key elements of cardiovascular nursing care at this level include the development, initiation, and maintenance of systems and processes that promote teamwork, effective communication, collaboration, efficiency, and patient satisfaction.

Cardiovascular nursing research is a well-developed aspect of the cardiovascular nursing role. Cardiovascular nursing research has broadened the scientific foundation of cardiovascular practice and continues to provide evidence of effective approaches and processes to quality cardiovascular nursing care.

Evolution of Cardiovascular Nursing Scope and Standards of Practice

The first scope and standards for cardiovascular nursing were developed and published in 1975 in collaboration with the American Heart Association (AHA) and updated in 1981. In 1993, the American Nurses Association Council on Medical-Surgical Nursing Practice published *The Scope of Cardiac Rehabilitation Nursing Practice*. Since that time, the scope of practice of cardiovascular nursing has expanded dramatically, coinciding with the exponential growth of new evidence-based nursing science regarding cardiovascular disease epidemiology and pathophysiology across the life span, and its assessment, diagnosis, treatment, and outcomes. The 2008 *Cardiovascular Nursing: Scope and Standards of Practice* is available in Appendix A.

The cardiovascular nursing scope of practice statement initially included hospital-based care for individuals experiencing acute, chronic, and critical cardiovascular illnesses. It has since evolved to include prevention, risk modification, and care across the full spectrum of healthcare settings for those who are stable, those with unstable acute or chronic cardiovascular illness, those dependent on life-support devices, and those with major comorbidities that affect cardiovascular illness assessment, diagnosis, treatment, and outcomes. The current practice of cardiovascular nursing requires extensive clinical knowledge and expertise to provide highly specialized acute, chronic, critical, or end-of-life care to patients, whether they are hospitalized or reside in home, community-based, or hospice care settings. Cardiovascular nurses partner with patients, families, communities, and other healthcare providers to enhance self-care and community support, utilizing evidence-based, innovative models of symptom and disease management to improve patient outcomes. Cardiovascular nurses also play a critical role in facilitating safe patient transitions among care providers and settings.

The great complexity of cardiovascular disease and its many associated comorbidities creates crucial roles for cardiovascular nurses as caregivers, direct-care providers, coordinators, educators, administrators, case managers, and quality specialists who optimize patient outcomes associated with specific cardiovascular diagnoses. Cardiovascular nurses provide multiple and complex treatments, many of which are initiated or directed by nurses. To effectively care for this population, cardiovascular nurses must have additional in-depth knowledge of hematologic, pulmonary, sleep-disordered, renal, metabolic, and immunologic conditions.

Patient education content must be tailored to meet the self-care needs of patients with multiple medical and psychosocial conditions. The cardiovascular nurse must be prepared to teach patients and families about diverse topics ranging from health promotion and disease prevention to end-of-life symptom management. Patient education topics include both prevention and risk reduction strategies (such as diet, exercise, and activity recommendations), as well as disease management topics focused on treatments, medications, complementary and alternative therapies, and diagnostic tests. In addition to this type of factual content, patient self-management skills and self-efficacy behaviors have to be assessed and incorporated in educational programs to reduce health risks and improve disease management success.

Ultimately, patients and caregivers need to be able to manage the cardiovascular condition and common symptoms, to recognize indicators of declining function, and to understand when to seek assistance from healthcare providers. As the catalyst for optimizing patient management and self-care, cardiovascular nurses must acknowledge cultural differences and incorporate patient preferences in order to ensure a mutually acceptable plan of care.

A cardiovascular nurse demonstrates a strong interest in the population, a quest for knowledge, and a desire to increase professional competence in this specialty. The term *cardiovascular nurse* signifies the expectation of a level of cardiovascular care knowledge (basic or advanced) and skills related to the patient's needs or the care setting. This knowledge and these skills entail synthesis of data, selection of evidence-based interventions, delivery of care, and evaluation of care delivery that ultimately help individuals or groups attain, maintain, or restore cardiovascular health, or meet a peaceful death.

Many professional organizations serve the educational and professional needs of cardiovascular nurses. This revised cardiovascular nursing scope and standards document continues to describe cardiovascular nursing practice based on the participation and contribution of numerous nursing organizations whose constituency includes cardiovascular nurses. (Summary descriptions and hyperlinks to the websites of these organizations appear in Appendix B.) This document will continue to be the foundation for cardiovascular nursing and will require regularly scheduled periodic assessment and evaluation to consistently represent the current state of the art and science for cardiovascular nursing practice.

Practice Characteristics for Cardiovascular Nursing

Cardiovascular care is collaborative in nature. Cardiovascular nurses partner with physicians, licensed independent providers, and many other healthcare team members in a wide range of practice settings, including acute care, skilled nursing and rehabilitation facilities, and home settings. An essential nursing role in these settings is direct or indirect contact with individuals who have actual or potential cardiovascular disease. Cardiovascular nurses work at the bedside in acute care settings (emergency, perioperative, acute, progressive, and intensive care for children and adults), transplant programs, cardiac rehabilitation, offices and clinics, community health, home care, and hospice or palliative care.

Many cardiovascular nurses work in practice settings such as family practice, pediatrics, internal medicine, and gerontology, with large patient populations who are aging and at risk for or have cardiovascular disease. Cardiovascular nurses work in other diverse settings as well, such as telemonitoring, cardiac catheterization, hybrid surgical/interventional and/or electrophysiology laboratories, noninvasive imaging, radiology, exercise testing, transplantation programs, and the pharmaceutical, information technology, and device industries. They also work in organizations to develop, implement, and evaluate care systems so that cardiovascular outcomes can be improved, as well as in professional societies and government organizations that develop and evaluate health policy.

Cardiovascular nurses provide specialized care by managing and directing clinics focused on cardiovascular risk reduction, anticoagulation, lipid management, hypertension management, heart failure, cardiac rhythm management, life-sustaining and lifesaving devices, infusion therapies, genetics counseling, peripartum care, and pediatric or adult congenital heart disease. Other cardiovascular nurses serve as educators and researchers in academic and practice settings. The nurse educators focus on the provision of prelicensure, graduate, and doctoral educational content to prepare the next generation of cardiovascular nurses. Cardiovascular nurse education, professional development, and advanced specialized clinical knowledge and skills must be commensurate with the nursing practice needs of the patient population and setting.

Educational Requirements for Cardiovascular Nurses

Cardiovascular nurses include licensed registered nurses (RN) and advanced practice registered nurses (clinical nurse specialists and nurse practitioners), nurse educators, administrators, case managers, quality specialists, and researchers. An RN, regardless of specialty, is licensed and authorized by a state, commonwealth, or territory to practice nursing. The RN is educationally prepared for competent practice at the novice level upon graduation from an accredited school of nursing and qualified by national examination for RN licensure.

The RN is educated in the science and art of nursing with the goal of helping individuals and groups attain, maintain, and restore health whenever possible. Experienced nurses may become proficient in one or more practice areas or roles and may focus on patient care in clinical nursing practice specialties, such as cardiovascular nursing. Specialized cardiovascular knowledge and experience may be acknowledged through an identified certification process, in which specific nursing educational requirements and demonstration of knowledge in cardiovascular nursing practice have been delineated and validated through certification. Examples are certifications from:

- American Association of Critical-Care Nurses (AACN) Certification Corporation; http://www.aacn.org/dm/mainpages/certificationhome. aspx

- American Association of Heart Failure Nurses Certification Board (AAHFN-CB); http://www.heartfailurecertification.com/home.php

- American Board of Cardiovascular Medicine Nursing Cardiovascular Nursing Exam; http://www.abcmcertification.com/

- American Nurses Credentialing Center (ANCC); http://www .nursecredentialing.org/Cardiac-VascularNursing

Cardiovascular nurses have a broad knowledge base in anatomy, physiology, pharmacology, pharmacogenomics, pharmacotherapeutics, nutrition, psychology, sociology, and developmental theory. Clinical competencies beyond those obtained in basic nursing education include assessment and management of cardiovascular conditions, education and counseling skills for comprehensive cardiovascular risk factor reduction, disease management, and encouragement of patients in a lifelong pattern of healthy living.

Competencies addressing the physiological, psychosocial, educational, cultural, and spiritual needs of patients living with chronic cardiovascular illness are essential, including skill in helping patients and families address end-of-life issues. Cardiovascular nurses must be knowledgeable of the principles of ethical practice and have resources available to evaluate the merits, risks, and social concerns of cardiovascular interventions. In addition, cardiovascular nurses must be educated in patient advocacy across the age spectrum and all healthcare environments.

The core of cardiovascular nursing practice centers on the use of critical thinking and decision making based on scientific information and theory combined with evidence-based guidelines related to cardiovascular care. In providing comprehensive care across the continuum from prevention to end of life, the cardiovascular nurse uses the nursing process to assess individual, family, group, and population needs to form an appropriate diagnosis, identify goals, design a mutually agreed-upon plan of care, coordinate and provide therapeutic interventions, document the care, and evaluate the action plan using an interprofessional case management approach.

Strong assessment skills are the foundation of quality cardiovascular nursing practice. These include both cardiac and vascular system assessment, in addition to assessment of all affected systems. Intensive knowledge of cardiovascular physiology, including the principles of electrophysiology and arrhythmia recognition, is necessary to accurately assess and appropriately respond to life-threatening conditions.

The evolution of knowledge and technologies has created complex equipment to monitor, evaluate, and manage cardiovascular patients and their disease. This equipment varies in complexity from simple diagnostic tools, such as the stethoscope and sphygmomanometer, to complex imaging systems that can diagnose a congenital heart defect before 20 weeks gestational age, facilitate reconstruction of damaged or defective hearts, and help clinicians guide catheters into coronary arteries. Patient monitoring systems likewise have evolved from simple bedside monitors of electrocardiograms to implantable devices to record and/or manage arrhythmias.

Cardiovascular nurses are monitoring critically ill patients remotely using telehealth electronic ICU technology. With the development of small chip microprocessors, cardiac rhythm management devices have become even more complex with the ability to monitor hemodynamic changes, analyze cardiac rhythms, and provide therapy for potentially fatal arrhythmias. Mechanical circulatory support devices have evolved from a bridge to cardiac transplantation to destination therapy for individuals with end-stage heart failure. As a result of the constant change in cardiac-related technologies, cardiovascular nurses must be committed to lifelong learning through completion of continuing education and training programs.

Many cardiovascular nurses learn to use and monitor the data from catheters and devices associated with medical, surgical, and preventive care for all ages of patients with cardiovascular conditions. Examples include pulmonary artery catheters, thoracic impedance or hemodynamic monitoring devices (internal or external systems), cardiac rhythm management devices, and mechanical circulatory support devices. With expertise in these advanced technologies, cardiovascular nurses can monitor the patient, evaluate the function of and manage information provided by the devices, and improve patient safety. This also includes assessment of patient responses and teaching patients and families about the temporary and long-term use of these devices.

A strong cardiovascular knowledge base is necessary for cardiovascular nursing administrators, researchers, case managers, quality specialists, and educators who may not provide direct clinical care. The combination of cardiovascular disease management expertise with leadership and expertise in these other areas provides opportunities to positively impact the health and well-being of cardiovascular patients and improve patient outcomes.

Advanced Practice Registered Nurses in Cardiovascular Care

Registered nurses with graduate education and advanced specialized clinical knowledge and skills may be recognized by their licensure jurisdiction as advanced practice registered nurses (APRNs), including clinical nurse specialists (CNSs) and nurse practitioners (NPs). See the 2008 APRN Consensus Model for details about APRN preparation as an NP or CNS (http://nursingworld.org/consensusmodel). These APRNs demonstrate a greater depth and breadth of nursing knowledge, data synthesis, advanced nursing skills, and significant autonomy.

NPs specializing in cardiovascular care require expanded knowledge and skills to provide expert care to individuals, groups, or populations at risk for or diagnosed with cardiovascular disease. They conduct comprehensive assessments and promote health and prevention of cardiovascular injury and disease. An NP specializing in cardiovascular care develops differential diagnoses, orders tests and procedures, performs physical examinations, interprets diagnostic and laboratory tests, makes diagnoses, and prescribes pharmacologic and nonpharmacologic therapies for the management and treatment of acute and chronic cardiovascular illness and disease.

NPs specializing in cardiovascular care practice in areas and with patient populations that are consistent with their education and practice experience, providing evidence-based health and medical care in primary, acute, and long-term settings. Practice models continue to evolve with the development and implementation of the *Consensus Model for APRN Regulation: Licensure, Accreditation, Certification, and Education* (2008) and changing state licensure and practice regulations. These models include NPs specializing in cardiovascular care who are in independent or both autonomous and collaborative practice with other healthcare professionals to treat and manage cardiovascular health problems. These APRNs promote cardiovascular health and disease prevention through patient and community education, advocating for heart-healthy lifestyles, performing cardiovascular risk assessments, and implementing risk factor modifications. These NPs may serve in a variety of nonclinical roles as managers, researchers, consultants, and patient advocates.

CNSs specializing in cardiovascular care are clinical experts in evidence-based cardiovascular nursing practice, treating and managing the health problems of cardiovascular patients and populations. CNSs integrate knowledge of disease and medical conditions into the assessment, diagnosis, and treatment of patients' cardiovascular illnesses in their practice. These APRNs also work collaboratively with other members of the healthcare team.

CNSs specializing in cardiovascular care design, implement, and evaluate both patient-specific and population-based programs of care, and provide leadership in advancing the practice of cardiovascular nursing to achieve quality and cost-effective patient outcomes. They lead interprofessional groups in designing and implementing innovative alternative solutions that address systems and patient care issues.

As direct care providers, CNSs specializing in cardiovascular care conduct comprehensive health assessments, develop differential diagnoses, and have prescriptive authority in accordance with state regulatory language, which allows them to prescribe pharmacologic and nonpharmacologic agents and treatments for the management of acute and chronic cardiovascular illness and disease. These CNSs serve as patient advocates and educators. They provide expert consultation and education to healthcare providers, and conduct and interpret research to improve practices and enhance patient outcomes.

Continuing Professional Development and Lifelong Learning for Cardiovascular Nurses

Cardiovascular nursing professional development is a lifelong process of active participation by the cardiovascular registered nurse or advanced practice registered nurse in learning experiences to acquire and maintain competence, enhance professional practice, and achieve career goals. Cardiovascular nursing professional development begins with the basic academic nursing preparation and continues throughout the professional life of the cardiovascular nurse.

Lifelong learning, which is the obligation and responsibility of all nurses, is expected and necessary to maintain and increase competence in cardiovascular nursing practice. Competence is essential to the provision of safe, quality health care to cardiovascular patients and ensures that the nurse can safely perform in a changing healthcare environment. Competence is the hallmark

of professionalism and is a means by which a professional is held accountable to society. Competence is reflected in the nurse's ability to use her or
his knowledge, skill, judgment, abilities, values, and beliefs to deliver quality
care to cardiovascular patients in a variety of situations and practice settings.
All cardiovascular patients should expect to receive care from cardiovascular
nurses who maintain professional nursing competence.

Cardiovascular nursing professional development encompasses the domains
of academic education, continuing education, and staff professional development.
Academic education consists of courses taken for credit in an institution of higher
education that may or may not lead to a degree, completion of a certification
program, or individual coursework taken to update oneself in the cardiovascular
specialty. Continuing education comprises a systematic professional learning
experience designed to augment the knowledge, skills, and abilities of the nurse,
thereby enriching the nurse's contribution to quality health care. Continuing
education can be part of a formal academic program, part of staff professional
development, or study for the purpose of enhancing cardiovascular nursing
practice. Staff professional development is the systematic process of assessment,
planning, education, and evaluation that enhances the performance or professional growth of the nurse within an organization. Staff professional development
can include continuing education and academic education programs.

Evidence-Based Practice and Research in Cardiovascular Nursing

The foundation of knowledge for cardiovascular nursing is embedded in
an academic nursing curriculum. The practice of cardiovascular nursing is
evidence-based and incorporates the continuous process of lifelong learning.
Demonstration of competence in practice is reflected in a practitioner's ability to continuously add to his or her knowledge and skills as the understanding of cardiovascular pathophysiology, management, and therapeutic targets
evolves. The science that guides practice is ever changing and based on rigor-
ous research. The source of evidence arises from many disciplines, including
nursing, medicine, psychology, and epidemiology, to name a few.

Cardiovascular nurses must rely on evolving knowledge that is often summa-
rized and presented in practice guidelines to help guide daily care of patients.
Guidelines offer recommendations, but cardiovascular nurses must evaluate
each individual within the context of the disease, and consider the impact
of psychosocial, economic, cultural, and other influences when considering

application of the guidelines. Patient preferences are respected in the joint patient-clinician plan of care.

The evolution of scientific knowledge is a result of research. Cardiovascular nurses develop, conduct, participate in, and evaluate research. Additionally, they participate in the delivery of care directed by these findings. They are scientists, clinical researchers, and clinicians who continue to add to the evolving literature about cardiovascular disease. The focus of cardiovascular nurses on the patient, family, and community provides a unique perspective on the delivery of care, and their research in these areas adds context and dimension to our understanding of cardiovascular disease and the impact of the disease on the patient, family, community, and healthcare providers.

Ethics in Cardiovascular Nursing

The ethical tradition of nursing continues to be self-reflective, enduring, and distinctive. Cardiovascular nurses recognize that they have ethical obligations to their patients, the profession, and their colleagues, as well as to the community. Ethics is a fundamental and integral component of cardiovascular nursing. The requisite for cardiovascular health care is universal, transcending all individual differences.

Cardiovascular nursing encompasses the prevention of cardiovascular illness; the alleviation of suffering from cardiovascular conditions; and the protection, promotion, and restoration of cardiovascular health. The cardiovascular nurse establishes relationships and delivers nursing care to patients and their families with respect for human dignity, the patient's right to self-determination, privacy, and confidentiality.

Across the life span, patients experience deteriorating cardiovascular-related conditions and other terminal illnesses. Requests for withdrawal or refusal of cardiovascular interventions from patients or their surrogates can be expected to increase and may produce conflict between competing ethical principles to respect patient autonomy, on the one hand, and to promote patient well-being (beneficence) and avoid harm (nonmaleficence), on the other. The cardiovascular nurse delivers nursing care without prejudice or bias and with respect for human needs and values.

ANA's *Code of Ethics for Nurses with Interpretive Statements* (2015) (the Code) makes explicit the primary goals, values, and obligations of the profession. The cardiovascular nurse recognizes, upholds, and promotes the values and beliefs described in the Code. Cardiovascular disease is complex, and its management can create complex ethical issues. The following content lists the nine provisions stated in the Code, followed by select examples of how cardiovascular nurses integrate and demonstrate the application of the provisions within their specialty practice. The vignettes reflect the complexity of cardiovascular patients, their care needs, and the cardiovascular nurse's associated decision making. Provisions 1, 2, and 3 are integrated in the first examples describing cardiovascular nursing care of an older adult and a pediatric patient.

Provision 1. The nurse practices with compassion and respect for the inherent dignity, worth, and uniqueness of every person.

Provision 2. The nurse's primary commitment is to the patient, whether an individual, family, group, community, or population.

Provision 3. The nurse promotes, advocates for, and protects the rights, health, and safety of the patient.

Older Adult Patient

Since the introduction of pacemakers (PMs) in 1958 and implantable cardioverter defibrillators (ICDs) in 1980, it has been well documented that these devices save and extend lives. As the indications for device therapy expand, the population of patients with devices continues to grow. More patients have devices, which increases the likelihood that the cardiovascular nurse device specialist will be faced with a request for device deactivation at the end of life.

A 71-year-old male with a past medical history of cardiomyopathy, New York Heart Association (NYHA) Functional Class III, had an ICD implanted in 2007 for clinical ventricular tachycardia. In 2012, the device was upgraded to a cardiac resynchronization defibrillator. His last high-voltage therapy for clinical ventricular tachycardia was in 2013. He is currently on optimal medical therapy for heart failure and anti-arrhythmic drug therapy.

Within the past 6 months, his health has progressively deteriorated and he reports severe lightheadedness, has been markedly hypotensive, and has recurrent, tense ascites. The healthcare team at the advanced heart failure clinic has stated that he is not a candidate for a left-ventricular assist device or transplant. After a lengthy discussion with the patient's healthcare team, the patient and family met and decided to take the patient home with home hospice and requested deactivation of the ICD.

According to Provisions 1, 2, and 3, it is ethical for the cardiovascular nurse device specialist to deactivate the ICD. The primary ethical principle supporting withdrawal of life-sustaining therapy is respect for the patient's autonomy and the patient's right to self-determination. The patient has the right to redefine the goals of care from treatment to symptom management that promotes comfort at the end of life. The patient can request withdrawal of unwanted medical interventions even if doing so results in death.

Pediatric Patient

Similarly, Provisions 1, 2, and 3 of the Code provide guidance for cardiovascular nurses in the care of fetuses, babies, children, and adults with congenital heart disease (CHD) through all phases of care after that diagnosis is confirmed. One of every 125 babies is born with congenital heart disease. Using echocardiogram technology, CHD may be identified as early as 12 to 15 weeks gestation. Other defects are identified within the first hours or weeks of life. Approximately 15% of these babies require complex, open-heart surgery within their first week of life (CDC, n.d.).

The parents and caregivers of these babies are faced with many complex ethical decisions that start at the time of diagnosis. Diagnosis at an early gestational age allows for therapeutic abortions. The complex anatomy of some babies may preclude surgical repair, leaving the parents the choice of heart transplantation, often in a city or state miles from their home, or comfort care. Postoperative surgical problems or unforeseen comorbidities may lead caregivers to offer withdrawal of life support and symptom management to promote comfort at the end of life.

Complex congenital heart disease was diagnosed in Baby A by a fetal echocardiogram at 16 weeks gestation. Baby A is the result of several months of advanced infertility management. At the same time, a significant chromosomal abnormality was identified by blood analysis. The baby's cardiac diagnosis necessitated delivery in a center several hundred miles from the couple's home, and open-heart surgery would be needed within the first few days of the baby's life. Ultimately, after several complex procedures and unsuccessful interventions, care providers advised that life-support measures be withdrawn, resulting in the death of the infant while being held in his parents' arms.

In this case the parents faced several points of critical decision making. At each point the cardiovascular nurse worked within the provisions of the *Code of Ethics* and with the family to "support the health, safety, and rights of the patient."

Provision 4. The nurse has authority, accountability, and responsibility for nursing practice; makes decisions; and takes action consistent with the obligation to promote health and provide optimal care.

A cardiac intensive care unit has a full census with six complex patients, including several who are from the cardiac surgical intensive care unit. Two patients are stable following acute myocardial infarction. One patient is one day postoperative after four-vessel coronary artery bypass graft (CABG) and has recently been extubated. Two patients are postoperative for destination left ventricular assist device (LVAD) placement: one is stable on day 2 and the other is two weeks postoperative and bleeding. The sixth is a 35-year-old male with an acute ST-segment myocardial infarction (STEMI) who is in cardiogenic shock.

The charge nurse makes assignments based on both the knowledge level and skills of the staff, as well as their ability to interact with the patients and their families. The charge nurse assigns the newer RNs to the stable patients (post-CABG and destination LVAD). The less stable patients are assigned to the more experienced nurses. The patient with an LVAD having complications and the young patient with a STEMI are each taken care of by experienced nurses who have worked with the palliative care team and have demonstrated a great deal of empathy with patients and families as they consider possible end-of-life decisions.

The staffing decisions made by this charge nurse reflect a decision-making process that is founded in Provision 4 as the obligation to provide optimal nursing care. Considering the needs of the patients and the attributes of each staff member will ensure that all of the patients' needs can be met.

Provision 5. The nurse owes the same duties to self as others, including the responsibility to promote health and safety, preserve wholeness of character and integrity, maintain competence, and continue personal and professional growth.

This provision addresses the need of the nurse to think of practice encounters in a way not represented in other provisions. The five components of this provision are often interrelated and complex.

In this provision the nurse performs a self-evaluation of learning needs to maintain safe and competent practice, as well as professional growth. This type of introspection may lead to seeking certification when it is not mandated by licensure or employer. Professional growth may include seeking opportunities to serve on committees at the place of employment, reading articles related to professional issues, or volunteering for a professional nursing organization.

This provision also addresses self-respect and preservation of integrity, which are important in preventing moral distress. Jameton (1984) described *moral distress* as a situation in which the person knows the appropriate action but is inhibited or constrained from taking it. The conflict may be related to inability to control factors in the work environment or fear of upsetting coworkers or family members. In recent years, the prevention of moral distress has been the focus of much nursing research, as it can result in nurses leaving the workplace.

Jayne is a 44-year-old woman with American Heart Association (AHA) Stage D heart failure due to adriamycin therapy for breast cancer. She is on guideline-directed medical therapies. Now Jayne is being considered for a ventricular assist device as destination therapy, even though her cancer could possibly return. The nurse recognizes that staff members are building false hope with this patient, who has professed that she is at peace. The nurse is timid around the Advanced Heart Failure team and afraid that they will not listen to the patient or her statements. The nurse wants the Advanced Heart Failure team to present palliative care as an option but is unable to articulate this recommendation. The nurse has experienced this several times before and is now frustrated and angry at work and expressing anxiety about going in to work most days. The nurse tells coworkers about plans to change jobs to find a happier work setting.

The cardiovascular unit's clinical nurse specialist recognizes that there has been a change in the staff nurse and plans a meeting to address the behavior change. The CNS recognizes that the nurse has avoided participating in rounds with the Advanced Heart Failure team and suspects that the nurse may be experiencing moral distress in the job. The CNS works with the nurse to identify the distress and provide strategies to help the nurse develop the skills needed to speak up within the group. Over time, the nurse becomes an active participant in the Advanced Heart Failure team's rounds.

Several approaches to reduce or prevent moral distress have been published. All focus on recognizing signs of moral distress and encouraging the nurse to voice concerns. The American Association of Critical-Care Nurses has developed a moral distress position statement and a tool kit to assist nurses in managing moral distress. Self-evaluation, planning a program to improve communication, and the support of management can uphold this ethical provision.

Provision 6. The nurse, through individual and collective effort, establishes, maintains, and improves the ethical environment of the work setting and conditions of employment that are conducive to safe, quality health care.

The complexity of healthcare systems, coupled with increasing financial constraints, creates a challenging environment for cardiovascular care. Increasing numbers of individuals, who are living longer with chronic and complex conditions, require the care of teams of healthcare professionals that span care settings. Ineffective teamwork, inadequate communication, and failure to engage patients and their families contribute to healthcare system failures. These shortcomings may result in inferior patient outcomes. Collaborative, interprofessional practice environments that foster improved patient outcomes, as well as nurse satisfaction, engagement, and retention, are essential.

Increasing interprofessional collaborative practice, improving care coordination, sharing decision-making processes, and refining transitional care are integral to improving patient care efficiency and effectiveness. Cardiovascular nurses have the responsibility to identify and address gaps in communication and care. The case study from Provision 5 can also be applied to this provision. Overcoming moral distress and finding a voice within the interprofessional team enabled the nurse to contribute to patient care and patient advocacy.

Provision 7. The nurse, in all roles and settings, advances the profession through research and scholarly inquiry, professional standards development, and the generation of both nursing and health policy.

Nursing practice is evolving as nursing takes on an ever-increasing and more complex role within health care and the society at large. Innovative and effective nursing curricula must be developed to prepare a cadre of competent and highly educated cardiovascular registered nurses. The rapid growth of critical care pathways, the use of integrated care delivery systems, and changes in professional roles and boundaries are continuously expanding nursing's scope of practice.

In an era of evidence-based practice, it is essential for cardiovascular nurses to incorporate a sequential layering of research throughout their clinical practices and to implement systemic intervention generated from new knowledge. It is vital for cardiovascular nurses to examine the relationship between pertinent theories and existing research and effectively build applicable clinical knowledge that facilitates analysis and translation of clinical findings into practical, actionable, and broadly applicable interventions.

Recent paradigm shifts in ways of understanding and explaining human experience mean that more fitting approaches to understanding and representing knowledge have come to be accepted within the scientific community. New paradigms of research processes include cause and effect, outcome-driven clinical pathways, and measurement of variance. It is imperative for cardiovascular nurses to be critically reflective.

The contribution and engagement of cardiovascular nurses in research enables successful translation of meaningful clinical outcomes from "bench to bedside." The benchmarks of cardiovascular nurses' involvement in translational research includes patients living to their highest potential and dissemination of evidence-based care into clinical practice. This allows nurse scientists to lead or be scientific members of interprofessional teams in a wide range of clinical and translational research projects.

Nurses review ethical principles and standards while conducting research to advance nursing science and the profession. Indeed, it is crucial that the questions and the motivation for research determine the methodological approach, rather than the method, dictating the shape and nature of questions. The particular perspective that nurses take when engaging in the research process will depend on their rationale for conducting the research, whether for nursing practice, education, administration, or knowledge development. Nursing continues to evolve and advance its knowledge through scientific inquiry by integrating theory and practice.

Provision 8: The nurse collaborates with other health professionals and the public to protect human rights, promote health diplomacy, and reduce health disparities.

Cardiovascular nurses are in the forefront of collaboration with other professional health colleagues in creating, innovating, educating, and moving advances in health care forward in the public sector. On the local level, nurses provide public education through the healthcare system, the school system, the business community, faith community nursing, and by being involved with their employers, family, and friends.

Joining forces enables greater impact in finding solutions, improving access to care, and developing policy related to prevention and treatment of cardiovascular disease. Through lobbying to improve insurance coverage for pre-existing conditions on the national level, nurses have the opportunity to be members and volunteer with diverse professional organizations, which have the best interest of patient care in the forefront of their mission and vision. Professional healthcare organizations have been key in promoting legislation to protect, insure, and care for individuals at all levels of intervention and across the continuum from acute care to transitional care to the home. All of the nursing organizations represented in the development of this cardiovascular scope and standards document are examples of such professional groups.

Lastly, on the international level, in addition to being involved in international professional associations, the RN can assert knowledge and expertise through collaboration with colleagues from various countries, sharing of research and practice initiatives, networking at meetings, participating in educational venues, and sharing practice innovations. By having a joint voice with like professionals, those in cardiovascular specialty nursing practice can continue to be leaders in nursing care, across the globe.

Provision 9: The profession of nursing, collectively through its professional organizations, must articulate nursing values, maintain the integrity of the profession, and integrate principles of social justice into nursing and health policy.

Cardiovascular nurses are fortunate to have membership options in several cardiovascular nursing specialty, quality, safety, and other professional organizations with a mission and vision that focus on patient care. One example of nursing involvement and articulation of nursing values would be working within the professional organization's many committees and workgroups. Committees such as those on education, health and public policy, healthcare reform, public documents oversight, certification, advocacy, program planning, professional publications, membership, disease management, and outcome provide excellent opportunities for cardiovascular nurses to lead, be involved in, and initiate quality practice initiatives across the nation.

Public and political understanding have increased and action toward supporting cardiovascular healthcare initiatives has been accomplished through the joint lobbying efforts of many professional nursing and other organizations in federal sectors and within individual states. One specific initiative that has spanned several years has been securing coverage for appropriate cardiac rehabilitation for several cardiac diagnoses and some preventive programs for older adults. Coverage by the Centers for Medicare and Medicaid Services (CMS) and commercial insurance is now available. Knowledge of current coverage and coverage changes for pre-existing illness states, improved healthcare access, new therapies, and new technologies places cardiovascular nurses in strategic positions for leading quality patient care.

Future Considerations

A host of issues and trends in health care influence specialty nursing care for individuals and families at risk for or with cardiovascular health problems. The large number of aging Baby Boomers; pandemics of sedentary lifestyle, obesity, and diabetes; the longer survival of children and adults with congenital heart disease; and the sheer volume of people requiring cardiovascular care will have a significant impact on healthcare resources and demands for services.

New discoveries about the genetic and pathophysiologic origins of disease and how they interact with environment and lifestyle have added to our already vast knowledge, challenging the nursing profession to stay current in providing care, advocating for patient needs, and teaching patients and their families. Emerging science about novel risk factors that increase the probability of cardiovascular disease, along with new diagnostic tests, treatments, interventions, and advances in genomics and genetics, including pharmacogenomics, will shape treatment choices in the future. Cardiovascular nurses are challenged to engage in lifelong learning to keep abreast of the rapidly developing science and to provide evidence-based nursing care. The translation of new knowledge and evidence into practice must be accelerated.

Significant and complex challenges to nurses anticipating patient healthcare needs are growing because of:

- Mandates for shortened length of stay

- Readmission management

- Sicker patients at discharge

- Lack of social support

- Too few or no caregivers

- Limited healthcare coverage and insurance resources

- Medical homes

- Patient-centered care

Emerging technologies intended to improve quality of life or prolong life, and those that require 24-hour care of patients, across the continuum, also challenge cardiovascular nurses to expand their creative thinking, in ways they may not have been challenged previously. The explosion of new information has heightened the necessity for and importance of using evidence in providing care and counseling for patients about their therapeutic options. Thus, maintaining current knowledge in this era of evidence-based practice is both challenging and essential.

A variety of issues related to the current nursing workforce and work environments warrant attention in planning for future cardiovascular health care. The continued projection of a nursing shortage, intensified by the aging of the nursing workforce, is well documented. Work environments must be transformed to retain experienced cardiovascular nurses.

Cardiovascular nurses must be involved in decisions related to creating patient care systems and healthy work environments. Continued efforts and funding to support nursing education are also essential to ensure adequate numbers of knowledgeable and competent cardiovascular nurses. New specialized healthcare provider roles increase the risk of fragmented, discontinuous care and poor communication, resulting in poor patient outcomes. The leadership of the cardiovascular nurse with enhanced skills in interdisciplinary communication and collaboration will be required to ensure patient safety and coordination of care.

Projected shortages of primary care physicians and changes in medical education provide opportunities for advanced practice registered nurses to fill the gap. Advanced practice registered nurses are also integral stakeholders in efforts to promote and improve interprofessional communication, interpret and accelerate the application of evidence to patient care, conduct research, and improve outcomes of care. Cardiovascular nurses encounter many new leadership opportunities in safety and quality initiatives, evidence-based practice, bench-to-bedside translational research, and other areas of emerging care. Changes in the healthcare environment provide an opportunity for registered nurses to collaborate with APRNs, physicians, and healthcare executives to reconfigure care systems and develop structures and processes that promote evidence-based practice.

Issues specific to care environments, including technology, workforce safety, and patient transitions, raise new challenges and opportunities. As the rate of technological advances increases, cardiovascular nurses need to be competent in the application and evaluation of technology; this includes incorporation of ethical decisions in the use of this technology. Additionally, critical thinking skills are required in knowing when to introduce palliative care for patient symptom management, comfort, safety, and quality of life, as well as in facilitating the transition to hospice care, when indicated. The incidence of adverse events and medical errors in all healthcare settings mandates a continued emphasis on safety and quality initiatives in caring for patients with cardiovascular healthcare needs.

Fragmentation of care contributes to a greater need for nurses to be able to provide seamless care and excellent communication as patients move between acute care, transitional care, community, and home settings. The shift of hospital-based therapies to ambulatory and home care settings requires a competent and knowledgeable nursing workforce, regardless of the setting where patients receive care. Telehealth technologies, which help nurses to assess, monitor, and treat patients remotely, require technological expertise, knowledge of transitional care issues, and vigilance to ensure continuing communication with patients and families about their health needs.

The growing number of infants and older adults with complex cardiovascular disease, combined with the complications of comorbidities and shortened hospital stays, will require cardiovascular nurses to address the complexities involved in the transition of patients across care settings. Increased communication between ambulatory and home-based care providers, improved discharge planning, and better training of families and caregivers to manage illness and appropriately access the healthcare system are needed.

The complexity of the healthcare system remains a challenge for many individuals and families who desire a more active role in decision making about health. Self-care and increased healthcare consumerism provide nurses with unique opportunities to influence outcomes. The healthcare needs of underserved and increasingly ethnically diverse populations present both opportunities and responsibilities for nurses. Quality of life, and how it affects patients' decisions about new therapies, is an important consideration, as are the knowledge, skills, and emotions of the family or caregiver. Advances in science, and increased patient longevity, afford nurses even greater opportunity to influence target audiences at multiple points across the life span. Emphasis on the patient's personal responsibility for improving health can foster stronger partnerships with healthcare decision makers considering various treatment options. Incorporating integrated therapies into care across the continuum has begun to be, and will continue to be, an integral part of nursing care responsibilities.

Initiatives in health promotion and disease prevention continue to be underfunded by insurance companies in most healthcare systems. The need to justify costly health care with improved outcomes has renewed the focus on prevention. However, standardized coding systems downplay interdisciplinary efforts, resulting in decreased reimbursement for such efforts and limiting innovation to meet these goals. Increasing financial burdens on consumers, employers, and government resources are providing opportunities for nurses to become part of future solutions.

Given the prevalence of people who are living with chronic, preventable cardiovascular conditions, cardiovascular nurses are in a unique position to create culturally relevant programs for individuals and communities. Prevention of cardiovascular disease starts in infancy. Educating people to make healthy lifestyle choices to avoid obesity, eliminate the use of all forms of tobacco, be more active, and eat better can significantly reduce morbidity and mortality associated with cardiovascular disease. Cardiovascular nurses need to be role models and demonstrate emerging knowledge of how successful behavioral change happens, as they lead patients to adopt healthier lifestyles.

The healthcare needs of underserved and ethnically diverse populations present both opportunities and responsibilities for nurses. Registered nurses with expertise in physiology, medicine, and behavioral change contribute to improvements in the health of individuals and families. Cardiovascular nurses bring unique knowledge, skills, and expertise that can be used to create innovative programs for improving the health of patients, families, and communities. Together, this competent and caring nursing workforce has the knowledge and expertise needed to care for the nearly 80 million people who are living with cardiovascular disease in the United States.

This current scope and standards publication for cardiovascular nursing provides the foundation for sound cardiovascular nursing practice. It is necessarily a living document, which will be continually updated as the understanding and management of cardiovascular disease advance.

Standards of Cardiovascular Nursing Practice

Significance of Standards

The Standards of Professional Nursing Practice are authoritative statements of the duties that all registered nurses, regardless of role, population, or specialty, are expected to perform competently. The standards published herein may be utilized as evidence of the standard of care, with the understanding that application of the standards is context dependent. The standards are subject to change with the dynamics of the nursing profession, as new patterns of professional practice are developed and accepted by the nursing profession and the public. In addition, specific conditions and clinical circumstances may also affect the application of the standards at a given time (e.g., during a natural disaster). The standards are subject to formal, periodic review and revision.

The competencies that accompany each standard may be evidence of compliance with the corresponding standard. The list of competencies is not exhaustive. Whether a particular standard or competency applies depends upon the circumstances.

Standards of Practice for Cardiovascular Nursing

Standard 1. Assessment

The cardiovascular registered nurse collects comprehensive data pertinent to the patient's health and/or the situation.

COMPETENCIES

The cardiovascular registered nurse:

- Collects comprehensive data including, but not limited to, physical, functional, psychosocial, emotional, cognitive, sexual, cultural, age-related, environmental, spiritual/transpersonal, and economic assessments in a systematic and ongoing process while honoring the uniqueness of the person regardless of age and across all settings.

- Applies appropriate cardiovascular expertise and knowledge to data collection in caring for patients with cardiovascular disease.

- Elicits the patient's values, preferences, expressed needs, and knowledge of the healthcare situation.

- Involves the patients, family, and other healthcare providers, as appropriate, in holistic data collection.

- Identifies barriers (e.g., psychosocial, literacy, financial, cultural) to effective communication and education and makes appropriate adaptations.

- Recognizes the impact of personal attitudes, values, and beliefs on the performance of nursing care.

- Assesses family dynamics and impact on patient health and wellness.

- Prioritizes data collection based on the patient's immediate condition, or the anticipated needs of the patient or situation.

- Uses appropriate evidence-based assessment techniques, instruments, and tools.

- Synthesizes available data, information, and knowledge relevant to the situation to identify patterns and variances.

- Applies ethical, legal, and privacy guidelines and policies to the collection, maintenance, use, and dissemination of data and information.

- Recognizes the patient as the authority on his or her own health by honoring the patient's care preferences.

- Documents relevant data in a retrievable format.

ADDITIONAL COMPETENCIES FOR THE APRN

The advanced practice registered nurse:

- Initiates and interprets diagnostic tests and procedures relevant to the patient's current status.

- Assesses the effect of interactions among individuals, family, community, and social systems on health and illness.

Standard 2. Diagnosis

The cardiovascular registered nurse analyzes the assessment data to determine the diagnoses or the issues.

COMPETENCIES

The cardiovascular registered nurse:

- Derives the diagnoses or issues from assessment data.

- Validates the diagnoses or issues with the patient, family, and other healthcare providers when possible and appropriate.

- Identifies actual or potential risks to the patient's health and safety or barriers to education or health, which may include, but are not limited to, interpersonal, systematic, or environmental circumstances.

- Uses standardized classification systems and clinical decision support tools, when available, in identifying diagnoses.

- Documents diagnoses or issues in a manner that facilitates the determination of the expected outcomes and plan.

ADDITIONAL COMPETENCIES FOR THE APRN

The advanced practice registered nurse:

- Systematically compares and contrasts clinical findings with normal and abnormal variations and developmental events in formulating a differential diagnosis.

- Applies appropriate advanced cardiovascular knowledge and expertise to the diagnostic process when caring for patients with cardiovascular disease.

- Utilizes complex data and information obtained during interview, examination, and diagnostic processes in identifying diagnoses.

- Facilitates staff development and maintenance of competence in the diagnostic process for cardiovascular disease.

Standard 3. Outcomes Identification

The cardiovascular registered nurse identifies expected outcomes for a plan individualized to the patient and the situation.

COMPETENCIES

The cardiovascular registered nurse:

- Involves the patients, family, healthcare providers, and others in formulating expected outcomes when possible and appropriate.

- Derives culturally appropriate expected outcomes from the diagnoses.

- Considers associated current scientific evidence, risks, benefits, costs, expected trajectory of the condition, and clinical expertise when formulating expected outcomes.

- Derives outcomes that enhance self-care as appropriate for the patient and/or family.

- Defines expected outcomes in terms of the patient's preferences, culture, values, and ethical values.

- Includes a time estimate for the attainment of expected outcomes.

- Develops expected outcomes that facilitate continuity of care.

- Modifies expected outcomes according to changes in the status of the patient or evaluation of the situation.

- Documents expected outcomes as measurable goals.

ADDITIONAL COMPETENCIES FOR THE APRN

The advanced practice registered nurse:

- Identifies expected outcomes that incorporate scientific evidence and are achievable through implementation of evidence-based practices.

- Identifies expected outcomes that incorporate cost and clinical effectiveness, patient satisfaction, and continuity and consistency across providers and care settings.

- Differentiates outcomes that require care process interventions from those that require system-level interventions.

Standard 4. Planning

The cardiovascular registered nurse develops a plan that prescribes strategies and alternatives to attain expected outcomes.

COMPETENCIES

The cardiovascular registered nurse:

- Develops an individualized plan, in partnership with the patient, family, and others, that considers the patient's characteristics or situation, including, but not limited to, values, beliefs, spiritual and health practices, preferences, choices, developmental level, coping style, culture and environment, and available technology.

- Establishes plan priorities with the patient, family, and others as appropriate.

- Applies cardiovascular expertise and knowledge in the planning of care for patients with cardiovascular disease.

- Includes strategies in the plan that address each of the identified diagnoses or issues. These strategies may include, but are not limited to, strategies for:

  - Promotion and restoration of health,

  - Prevention of illness, injury, and disease,

  - The alleviation of suffering, and

  - Supportive care for those who are dying.

- Includes strategies for health and wholeness across the life span.

- Provides for continuity in the plan so that transitions in the care continuum are safe and effective.

- Incorporates an implementation pathway or timeline in the plan.

- Considers the economic impact of the plan on the patient, family, caregivers, or others.

- Integrates current scientific evidence, trends, and research.

- Utilizes the plan to provide direction to other members of the healthcare team.

- Explores practice settings and safe space and time for the nurse and the patient to explore suggested, potential, and alternative options.

- Defines the plan to reflect current statutes, rules and regulations, and standards.

- Modifies the plan according to ongoing assessment of the patient's response and other outcome indicators.

- Documents the plan in a manner that uses standardized language or recognized terminology.

ADDITIONAL COMPETENCIES FOR THE APRN

The advanced practice registered nurse:

- Identifies assessment strategies, diagnostic strategies, and therapeutic interventions that reflect current evidence, including data, research, literature, and expert clinical knowledge.

- Selects or designs strategies to meet the multifaceted needs of complex patients.

- Includes the synthesis of patients' values and beliefs regarding nursing and medical therapies in the plan.

- Leads the design and development of interprofessional processes to address the identified diagnosis or issue.

- Actively participates in the development and continuous improvement of systems that support the planning process.

Standard 5. Implementation

The cardiovascular registered nurse implements the identified plan.

COMPETENCIES

The cardiovascular registered nurse:

- Partners with the healthcare consumer, family, significant others, and caregivers as appropriate to implement the plan in a safe, realistic, and timely manner.

- Demonstrates caring behaviors toward patients, significant others, and groups of people receiving care.

- Utilizes technology to measure, record, and retrieve patient data, implement the nursing process, and enhance nursing practice.

- Utilizes evidence-based interventions and treatments specific to the diagnosis or problem.

- Provides holistic care that addresses the needs of diverse populations across the life span.

- Advocates for health care that is sensitive to the needs of culturally diverse populations.

- Applies appropriate cardiovascular expertise and knowledge in caring for healthcare consumers with major health problems in implementing the plan of care.

- Applies available healthcare technologies to maximize access and optimize outcomes for patients.

- Utilizes community resources and systems to implement the plan.

- Collaborates with nursing colleagues and other healthcare providers from diverse professional backgrounds to implement and integrate the plan.

- Accommodates different styles of learning and communication used by patients, families, and healthcare providers.

- Integrates traditional and complementary healthcare practices as appropriate.

- Implements the plan in a timely manner in accordance with patient safety goals.

- Promotes the patient's capacity for the optimal level of participation in self-care and problem solving.

- Documents implementation and any modifications, including changes or omissions, of the identified plan.

ADDITIONAL COMPETENCIES FOR THE APRN
The advanced practice registered nurse:

- Facilitates utilization of systems, organizations, and community resources to implement the plan.

- Supports collaboration with nursing and other colleagues to implement the plan.

- Incorporates new knowledge and strategies to initiate changes in nursing care practices if desired outcomes are not achieved.

- Assumes responsibility for safe and efficient implementation of the plan.

- Use advanced communication skills to promote relationships between nurses and patients, to provide a context for open discussion of the patient's experiences, and to improve patient outcomes.

- Actively participates in the development and continuous improvement of systems that support implementation of the plan.

Standard 5A. Coordination of Care

The cardiovascular registered nurse coordinates care delivery.

COMPETENCIES

The cardiovascular registered nurse:

- Organizes the components of the plan.

- Manages a patient's cardiovascular care so as to maximize independence and quality of life.

- Assists the patient to identify options for alternative care.

- Communicates with the patient, family, and healthcare system, including referring clinicians and community resources, during transitions in care.

- Advocates for the delivery of dignified and humane care by the interprofessional team.

- Documents the coordination of care.

ADDITIONAL COMPETENCIES FOR THE APRN

The advanced practice registered nurse:

- Provides leadership in the coordination of cardiovascular care with the interprofessional healthcare team for integrated delivery of patient care services.

- Synthesizes data and information to prescribe necessary system and community support measures, including modifications of surroundings.

Standard 5B. Health Teaching and Health Promotion

The cardiovascular registered nurse employs strategies to promote health and a safe environment.

COMPETENCIES

The cardiovascular registered nurse:

- Provides health teaching that addresses such topics as healthy lifestyles, risk-reducing behaviors, developmental needs, activities of daily living, preventive care, and maintenance of self-care.

- Uses health promotion and health teaching methods, including "teach back" strategies, appropriate to the situation and the patient's health literacy, values, beliefs, health practices, developmental level, learning needs, readiness and ability to learn, preferred learning style, language preference, spirituality, culture, and socioeconomic status.

- Seeks opportunities for feedback and evaluation of the effectiveness of the strategies used.

- Uses information technologies to communicate health promotion and disease prevention information to the patient in a variety of settings.

- Provides patients with information about intended effects and potential adverse effects of proposed therapies.

ADDITIONAL COMPETENCIES FOR THE APRN

The advanced practice registered nurse:

- Synthesizes empirical evidence on risk behaviors, learning theories, behavioral change theories, motivational theories, epidemiology, and other related theories and frameworks when designing health education information and programs.

- Conducts personalized health teaching and counseling that incorporates comparative effectiveness research recommendations.

- Utilizes a holistic humanistic approach based on experiential analysis of the psychosocial aspect to enhance the learning and teaching.

- Designs health information and patient education appropriate to the patient's developmental level, learning needs, readiness to learn, and cultural values and beliefs.

- Evaluates health information resources, such as the Internet and social media, in the area of practice for accuracy, readability, and comprehensibility, to help patients access quality health information.

- Engages consumer alliances and advocacy groups, as appropriate, in health teaching and health promotion activities.

- Provides anticipatory guidance to individuals, families, groups, and communities to promote health and prevent or reduce the risk of health problems.

Standard 5C. Consultation

The advanced practice registered nurse provides consultation to influence the identified plan, enhance the abilities of others, and effect change.

COMPETENCIES FOR THE APRN

The advanced practice registered nurse:

- Synthesizes clinical data, theoretical frameworks, and evidence when providing consultation.

- Facilitates the effectiveness of a consultation by involving the healthcare consumer, family, and other stakeholders in decision making and negotiating role responsibilities.

- Facilitates the effectiveness of a consultation by conducting research and disseminating research and evidence-based practice findings to enhance both psychosocial and clinical patient and population outcomes.

- Communicates consultation recommendations.

Standard 5D. Prescriptive Authority and Treatment

The advanced practice registered nurse uses prescriptive authority, procedures, referrals, treatments, and therapies, based on education, certification, credentialing, and APRN scope of practice, in accordance with state and federal laws and regulations.

COMPETENCIES FOR THE APRN

The advanced practice registered nurse:

- Prescribes evidence-based treatments, therapies, devices, and procedures considering the patient's comprehensive healthcare needs.

- Prescribes pharmacologic agents based on current knowledge of pharmacology, physiology, and pathophysiology.

- Prescribes specific pharmacologic agents or treatments based on clinical indicators, comparative effectiveness, the patient's status and needs, and the results of genetic, diagnostic, and laboratory tests.

- Performs invasive and noninvasive therapeutic and diagnostic procedures based on education, certification, and credentialing.

- Evaluates therapeutic and potential adverse effects of pharmacologic and nonpharmacologic treatments.

- Provides patients with information about intended effects and potential adverse effects of proposed prescriptive therapies.

- Provides information about costs and alternative treatments and procedures, as appropriate.

- Evaluates and incorporates complementary and alternative therapies into education and practice.

Standard 6. Evaluation

The cardiovascular registered nurse evaluates progress toward attainment of outcomes.

COMPETENCIES

The cardiovascular registered nurse:

- Conducts a systematic, ongoing, and criterion-based evaluation of the outcomes in relation to the structures and processes prescribed by the plan of care, the indicated timeline, and cardiovascular expertise and knowledge.

- Collaborates with the patient and others involved in the care or situation in the evaluation process.

- Evaluates, in partnership with the patient, the effectiveness of the planned strategies in relation to the patient's responses and attainment of the expected outcomes.

- Uses ongoing assessment data to revise the diagnoses, outcomes, plan, and implementation as needed.

- Disseminates the results to the patient, family, and others involved, in accordance with federal and state regulations.

- Participates in assessing and assuring the responsible and appropriate use of interventions in order to minimize unwarranted or unwanted treatment and patient suffering.

- Documents the results of the evaluation.

ADDITIONAL COMPETENCIES FOR THE APRN

The advanced practice registered nurse:

- Evaluates the accuracy of the diagnosis and the effectiveness of the interventions and other variables in relation to the patient's attainment of expected outcomes.

- Synthesizes the results of the evaluation to determine the effect of the plan on patients, families, groups, communities, and institutions.

- Adapts the plan of care for the trajectory of treatment according to evaluation of the patient's response.

- Uses the results of the evaluation to implement process or structural changes, including policy, procedure, or protocol revision, as appropriate.

Standards of Professional Performance for Cardiovascular Nursing

Standard 7. Ethics

The cardiovascular registered nurse practices ethically.

COMPETENCIES

The cardiovascular registered nurse:

- Uses *Code of Ethics for Nurses with Interpretive Statements* (ANA, 2015) to guide practice.

- Delivers care in a manner that preserves and protects patient autonomy, dignity, rights, values, and beliefs.

- Recognizes the centrality of the patient and family as core members of the healthcare team.

- Maintains patient confidentiality within legal and regulatory parameters.

- Assists patients, family, and caregivers in self-determination and informed decision making.

- Maintains a therapeutic and professional patient–nurse relationship within appropriate professional role boundaries.

- Contributes to resolving ethical issues involving patients, colleagues, community groups, systems, and other stakeholders.

- Takes appropriate action regarding instances of illegal, unethical, or inappropriate behavior that can endanger or jeopardize the best interests of the patient or situation.

- Advocates when appropriate to question healthcare practice when necessary for safety and quality improvement.

- Advocates for equitable patient care.

ADDITIONAL COMPETENCIES FOR THE APRN

The advanced practice registered nurse:

- Collaborates in interprofessional teams that address ethical risks, benefits, and outcomes.

- Leads interprofessional teams to address ethical issues, risks, benefits, and outcomes.

- Provides information on the risks, benefits, and outcomes of healthcare regimens to allow informed decision making by the patient, family, and caregivers, including informed consent and informed refusal.

Standard 8. Education

The cardiovascular registered nurse attains knowledge and competence that reflect current nursing practice.

COMPETENCIES

The cardiovascular registered nurse:

- Participates in ongoing educational activities related to appropriate knowledge bases and professional issues.

- Demonstrates a commitment to lifelong learning through self-reflection and inquiry to address learning and personal growth needs.

- Seeks experiences that reflect current practice to maintain knowledge, skills, abilities, and judgment in clinical practice or role performance.

- Acquires knowledge and skills appropriate to the role, population, specialty, setting, situation, innovations, and new technologies.

- Seeks formal and independent learning experiences to develop and maintain clinical and professional skills and knowledge.

- Identifies learning needs based on nursing knowledge, nursing roles, and the changing needs of the population.

- Participates in formal or informal consultations to address issues in nursing practice as an application of education and knowledge base.

- Shares educational findings, experiences, and ideas with peers.

- Contributes to a work environment that is conducive to the education of healthcare professionals.

- Maintains professional records that provide evidence of competence and lifelong learning.

- Shares expertise with nurses and other healthcare providers, individually or in groups (e.g., precepts students and new staff, provides unit in-service on new cardiovascular therapies and treatments, teaches continuing education classes, etc.).

ADDITIONAL COMPETENCIES FOR THE APRN

The advanced practice registered nurse:

- Uses current healthcare research findings and other evidence to expand clinical knowledge, skills, abilities, and judgment; to enhance role performance; and to increase knowledge of professional issues.

Standard 9. Evidence-Based Practice and Research

The cardiovascular registered nurse integrates evidence and research findings into practice.

COMPETENCIES

The cardiovascular registered nurse:

- Utilizes current evidence-based nursing knowledge, including research findings, to guide practice.

- Incorporates evidence when initiating changes in nursing practice.

- Participates, as appropriate to education level and position, in the formulation of evidence-based practice through research. Such activities may include:

  - Incorporating research as a basis for learning and evidence-based practice.

  - Identifying clinical problems and questions that are conducive to nursing research (patient care and nursing practice).

  - Participating in data collection (surveys, pilot projects, qualitative studies that describe the lived experience, and formal studies).

  - Participating in a formal committee or program.

  - Sharing personal or third-party research findings with colleagues and peers.

  - Conducting research, quality improvement, or evidence-based projects.

  - Critically analyzing and interpreting research for application to practice.

  - Using research findings in the development of policies, procedures, and standards of practice.

ADDITIONAL COMPETENCIES FOR THE APRN

The advanced practice registered nurse:

- Contributes to nursing knowledge by conducting or synthesizing research and other evidence that discovers, examines, and evaluates current practice, knowledge, theories, criteria, and creative approaches to improve healthcare outcomes.

- Promotes a climate of research and clinical inquiry.

- Disseminates research findings through activities such as presentations, publications, consultation, and journal clubs.

Standard 10. Quality of Practice

The cardiovascular registered nurse contributes to quality nursing practice.

COMPETENCIES

The cardiovascular registered nurse:

- Demonstrates quality by documenting the application of the nursing process in a responsible, accountable, and ethical manner.

- Uses creativity and innovation to enhance nursing care.

- Participates in quality improvement. Activities may include:

  - Identifying aspects of practice important for quality monitoring.

  - Using indicators to monitor quality, safety, and effectiveness of nursing practice.

  - Collecting data to monitor quality and effectiveness of nursing practice.

  - Analyzing quality data to identify opportunities for improving nursing practice.

  - Formulating recommendations to improve nursing practice or outcomes.

  - Implementing activities to enhance the quality of nursing practice.

  - Developing, implementing, and/or evaluating policies, procedures, and guidelines to improve the quality of practice.

  - Participating on and/or leading interprofessional teams to evaluate clinical care or health services.

  - Participating in and/or leading efforts to minimize costs and unnecessary duplication.

  - Identifying problems that occur in day-to-day work routines so as to correct process and workflow inefficiencies.

  - Analyzing factors related to quality, safety, and effectiveness.

- Analyzing organizational systems for barriers to quality patient outcomes.

- Implementing processes to remove or weaken barriers within organizational systems.

- Comparing outcome data to national cardiovascular core measures and other program assessment metrics.

ADDITIONAL COMPETENCIES FOR THE APRN

The advanced practice registered nurse:

- Provides leadership in the design and implementation of quality improvements.

- Designs innovations to effect change in practice and improve health outcomes.

- Evaluates the practice environment and quality of nursing care rendered in relation to existing evidence.

- Identifies opportunities for the generation and use of research and evidence.

- Obtains and maintains professional certification if it is available in the area of expertise.

- Uses the results of quality improvement to initiate changes in nursing practice and the healthcare delivery system.

Standard 11. Communication

The cardiovascular registered nurse communicates effectively in a variety of formats in all areas of practice.

COMPETENCIES

The cardiovascular registered nurse:

- Assesses communication format preferences of patients, families, and colleagues.*

- Assesses her or his own communication skills in encounters with patients, families, and colleagues.*

- Seeks continuous improvement of her or his own communication and conflict resolution skills.*

- Conveys information to patients, families, the interprofessional team, and others in communication formats that promote accuracy.

- Questions the rationale supporting care processes and decisions when they do not appear to be in the best interest of the patient.*

- Discloses observations or concerns related to hazards and errors in care or the practice environment to the appropriate level.

- Maintains communication with patient, families, and other providers to minimize risks associated with transfers and transitions in care delivery.

- Contributes her or his own professional perspective in discussions with the interprofessional team.

* BHE/MONE, 2006.

Standard 12. Leadership

The cardiovascular registered nurse demonstrates leadership in the practice setting and the profession.

COMPETENCIES

The cardiovascular registered nurse:

- Oversees the nursing care given by others while retaining accountability for the quality of care given to the patient.

- Supports the vision, associated goals, and plan to implement and measure progress of an individual patient or progress within the context of the healthcare organization.

- Demonstrates a commitment to continuous, lifelong learning and education for self and others.

- Mentors colleagues for the advancement of nursing practice, the profession, and quality health care.

- Treats colleagues with respect, trust, and dignity.*

- Develops communication and conflict resolution skills.

- Participates in professional organizations.

- Communicates effectively with the patient and colleagues.

- Seeks ways to advance nursing autonomy and accountability.*

- Participates in efforts to impact healthcare policy.

ADDITIONAL COMPETENCIES FOR THE APRN

The advanced practice registered nurse:

- Leads decision-making groups and organizations to improve the professional practice environment and patient outcomes.

- Provides direction to enhance the effectiveness of the interprofessional team.

---

* BHE/MONE, 2006.

- Promotes advanced practice nursing and role development by interpreting its role for patients, families, and others.

- Models expert practice to interprofessional team members and patients.

- Mentors colleagues in the acquisition of clinical knowledge, skills, abilities, and judgment.

Standard 13. Collaboration

The cardiovascular registered nurse collaborates with patient, family, and others in the conduct of nursing practice.

COMPETENCIES

The cardiovascular registered nurse:

- Partners with others to effect change and produce positive outcomes through the sharing of knowledge of the patient and/or situation.

- Communicates with the patient, the family, caregivers, and healthcare providers regarding patient care and the nurse's role in the provision of that care.

- Invites the contribution of the patient, family, caregiver, and team members in order to achieve optimal outcomes.

- Promotes conflict management and engagement.

- Participates in building consensus or resolving conflict in the context of care.

- Applies group process and negotiation techniques with patients and colleagues.

- Adheres to standards and applicable codes of conduct that govern behavior among peers and colleagues to create a work environment that promotes cooperation, respect, and trust.

- Cooperates in creating a documented plan, focused on outcomes and decisions related to care and delivery of services, that indicates communication with patients, families, and others.

- Engages in teamwork and team-building processes.

ADDITIONAL COMPETENCIES FOR THE APRN

The advanced practice registered nurse:

- Partners with others on the interprofessional team to enhance patient outcomes through integrated activities, such as education, consultation, management, technological development, or research opportunities.

- Creates a patient-centered interprofessional process with other members of the healthcare team.

- Leads in establishing, improving, and sustaining collaborative relationships to achieve safe, quality patient care.

- Documents plan-of-care communications, rationales for plan-of-care changes, and collaborative discussions to improve patient outcomes.

Standard 14. Professional Practice Evaluation

The cardiovascular registered nurse evaluates her or his own nursing practice in relation to professional practice standards and guidelines, relevant statutes, rules, and regulations.

COMPETENCIES

The cardiovascular registered nurse:

- Provides age-appropriate and developmentally appropriate care in a culturally and ethnically sensitive manner.

- Engages in self-evaluation of practice with emphasis on cardiovascular nursing on a regular basis, identifying areas of strength as well as areas in which professional growth would be beneficial.

- Obtains informal feedback regarding her or his own practice from patients, peers, professional colleagues, and others.

- Participates in peer review as appropriate.

- Takes action to achieve goals identified during the evaluation process.

- Provides the evidence for practice decisions and actions as part of the informal and formal evaluation processes.

- Interacts with cardiovascular practitioners, educators, peers, and colleagues to enhance her or his own professional nursing practice or role performance.

- Provides peers with formal or informal constructive feedback regarding their practice or role performance.

ADDITIONAL COMPETENCIES FOR THE APRN

The advanced practice registered nurse:

- Engages in a formal process seeking feedback regarding her or his own cardiovascular practice from patients, peers, professional colleagues, and others.

Standard 15. Resource Utilization

The cardiovascular registered nurse utilizes appropriate resources to plan and provide nursing services that are safe, effective, and financially responsible.

COMPETENCIES

The cardiovascular registered nurse:

- Assesses individual patient care needs and resources available to achieve desired outcomes.

- Identifies patient care needs, potential for harm, complexity of the task, and desired outcome when considering resource allocation.

- Delegates elements of care to appropriate healthcare workers in accordance with any applicable legal or policy parameters or principles.

- Identifies the evidence when evaluating resources.

- Advocates for resources, including technology, that enhance nursing practice.

- Modifies practice when necessary to promote positive interaction between patients, care providers, and technology.

- Assists the patient and family in identifying and securing appropriate services to address needs across the healthcare continuum.

- Assists the patient and family in factoring costs, risks, and benefits into decisions about treatment and care.

ADDITIONAL COMPETENCIES FOR THE APRN

The advanced practice registered nurse:

- Utilizes organizational and community resources to formulate interprofessional plans of care.

- Formulates innovative solutions for patient care problems that utilize resources effectively and maintain quality.

- Designs evaluation strategies that demonstrate cost effectiveness, cost benefit, and efficiency factors associated with nursing practice.

- Synthesizes clinical data and available resource options to avoid duplication of services.

- Evaluates factors related to patient preferences, safety, effectiveness, and cost when two or more practice options would result in the same expected patient outcomes.

- Assigns tasks or delegates care based on the needs of the patient and the knowledge and competence of the provider selected.

Standard 16. Environmental Health

The cardiovascular registered nurse practices in an environmentally safe and healthy manner.

COMPETENCIES

The cardiovascular registered nurse:

- Attains knowledge of environmental health concepts, such as implementing environmental health strategies.

- Promotes a practice environment that reduces environmental health risks for workers and patients.

- Assesses the practice environment for factors such as sound, odor, noise, and light that threaten health or interfere with health promotion.

- Advocates for the judicious and appropriate use of products in health care.

- Communicates environmental health risks and exposure reduction strategies to patients, families, colleagues, and communities.

- Utilizes scientific evidence to determine if a product or treatment is an environmental threat.

- Participates in strategies to promote healthy communities.

ADDITIONAL COMPETENCIES FOR THE APRN

The advanced practice registered nurse:

- Creates partnerships that promote sustainable environmental health policies and conditions.

- Analyzes the impact of social, political, and economic influences on the environment and human health exposures.

- Critically evaluates the manner in which environmental health issues are presented by the popular media.

- Advocates for implementation of environmental principles in nursing practice.

Glossary

cardiovascular nursing. Specialized nursing care focused on the optimization of cardiovascular health across the life span and in diverse practice settings. Cardiovascular nursing care includes education, prevention, detection, and treatment of cardiovascular disease in individuals, families, communities, and populations.

registered nurse. An individual who is licensed by a state agency to practice as a registered nurse.

Standards of Practice. Authoritative statements that describe a competent level of clinical nursing practice demonstrated through assessment, diagnosis, outcomes identification, planning, implementation, and evaluation.

Standards of Professional Performance. Authoritative statements that describe a competent level of behavior in the professional role.

References

American Heart Association (AHA). (2015). AHA statistical update: Heart disease and stroke statistics—2015 update. Available at http://circ.ahajournals.org/content/early/2014/12/18/CIR.0000000000000152.full.pdf+html

American Nurses Association. (2015). *Code of Ethics for Nurses with interpretive statements*. Silver Spring, MD: Nursesbooks.org.

Board of Higher Education & Massachusetts Organization of Nurse Executives (BHE/MONE). (2006). *Creativity and connections: Building the framework for the future of nursing education (Report from the Invitational Working Sessions, March 23–24, 2006)*. Burlington, MA: MONE. Available at http://www.mass.edu/nahi/documents/NursingCreativityAndConnections.pdf

Centers for Disease Control and Prevention (CDC). (n.d.). Congenital heart defects (CHDs). Available at http://www.cdc.gov/ncbddd/heartdefects/features/heartdefects-keyfindings2010.html

Consensus Model for APRN regulation: Licensure, accreditation, certification, and education. (2008). Available at http://nursingworld.org/consensusmodel

Healthy People 2020. Available at https://www.healthypeople.gov/

Jameton, A. (1984). *Nursing practice: The ethical issues*. Englewood Cliffs, NJ: Prentice-Hall.

Kavey, R. W., Simmons-Morton, D. G., & deJesus, J. M. (2011). Expert panel on integrated guidelines for cardiovascular health and risk reduction in children and adolescents: Summary report. *Pediatrics, 128*(Suppl. 5), S1–S44.

Musunuru, K., et al. (2015). *Basic concepts and potential applications of genetics and genomics for cardiovascular and stroke clinicians: A scientific statement from the American Heart Association*. Online publication before print January 1, 2015. Available at http://circgenetics.ahajournals.org/content/early/2015/01/05/HCG.0000000000000020

Appendix A.

Cardiovascular Nursing:
Scope and Standards
of Practice (2008)

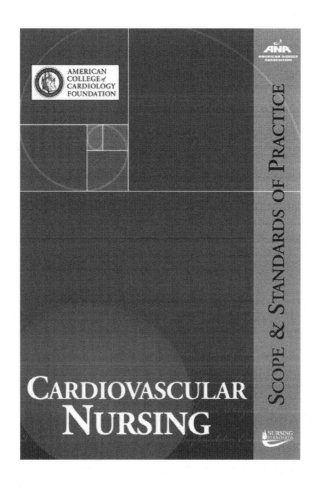

The content in this appendix is not current and is of historical significance only.

ACKNOWLEDGMENTS

This document was developed by a Task Force of Cardiovascular Nursing Organization Representatives whose collaborative efforts were vital to the development of a scope and standards for cardiovascular nursing that represents the diversity of practice today. The members of the task force gratefully acknowledge the support of the American College of Cardiology Foundation in facilitating the collaboration for this document. The Scope and Standards Task Force would like to give thanks to Carol J. Bickford, PhD, RN-BC, Senior Policy Fellow, Department of Nursing Practice and Economics, for her guidance in the development of the *Cardiovascular Nursing: Scope and Standards of Practice*.

Scope and Standards Task Force Members

Eileen Handberg, PhD, ARNP-BC, FAHA (Chair)
Nancy M. Albert PhD, CCNS, CCRN, CNA, FAHA
Angela P. Clark, PhD, RN, CNS, FAAN, FAHA
Paula Feeley-Coe, MSN, RN, CCTC
Jonni Cooper, PhD, MBA, BSN, CVRN
Kenneth A. Gorski, RN, RCIS, FSICP
Meg Gulanick, PhD, APRN, FAAN, FAHA
Melanie T. Gura, MSN, RN, CNS, FHRS, FAHA
Patricia A. Matula, MSN, RN
Robin E. Rembsburg, PhD, APRN-BC, FNGNA, FAAN
Barbara Riegel, DNSc, RN, CS, FAAN
Mary Rummell, MN, RN, CPNP, CNS
Kristen Sethares, PhD, RN
Julie Stanik-Hutt, PhD, ACNP, CCNS
Robin J. Trupp, PhD(c), MSN, ACNP-BC, CCRN, CCRC, FAHA
Kathleen K. Zarling, MS, APRN-BC, FAACVPR

The content in this appendix is not current and is of historical significance only.

Scope and Standards Reviewers

Douglas Beinborn, MA, BSN
Barbara J. Fletcher, MN, RN, FAHA, FAAN
Erika S. Froelicher, PhD, RN, FAAN, FAHA
Suzanne Hughes, MSN, RN, FAHA
Jane A. Linderbaum, MS, FNP
Kathleen McCauley, PhD, RN-BC, FAAN, FAHA
Ellen Strauss McErlean, MSN, RN, FAHA, CNS
Elizabeth Tong, MS, RN, CPNP, FAHA, FAAN

American College of Cardiology Foundation Staff Liaisons

Christina A. Chadwick, MSN, RN
Brenda Dorick-Miller, MSN, RN
Marcia Jackson, PhD

American Nurses Association (ANA) Staff

Carol J. Bickford, PhD, RN-BC—Content Editor
Yvonne Humes, MESA—Project Coordinator
Theresa Myers, JD—Legal Counsel

Endorsing Organizations

Descriptions and websites of these groups are in Appendix A, which begins on pg. 45.

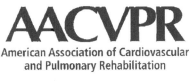

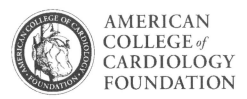

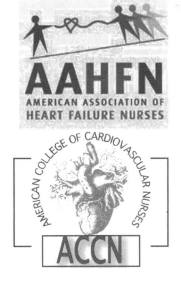

The content in this appendix is not current and is of historical significance only.

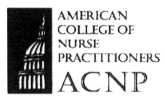

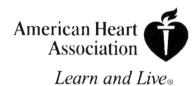

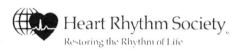

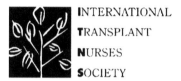

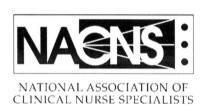

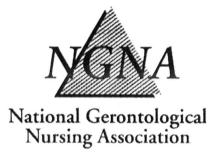

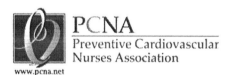

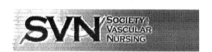

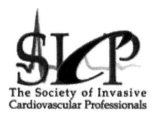

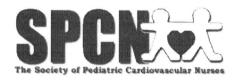

The content in this appendix is not current and is of historical significance only.

CONTENTS

The content in this appendix is not current and is of historical significance only.

The content in this appendix is not current and is of historical significance only.

INTRODUCTION

Cardiovascular disease is the primary cause of death and disability in men and women worldwide. Cardiovascular disease is responsible for over 36% of all deaths in America. Nearly 80 million adults in the United States are currently living with some form of cardiovascular disease. An estimated 37 million of these are 65 years or older. One out of every 85 babies is born with a congenital heart defect, which is now the major cause of birth-defect-related deaths. The number of people with severe congenital heart disease has risen by 85% in adults and by 22% in children over the past 15 years. Diseases of the cardiovascular system are responsible for much of the economic burden of health care in the United States and other developed countries. The estimated medical and disability cost for treatment of cardiovascular diseases in 2007 is $431 billion (AHA 2007).

Over the past 60 years, nurses have been key members of teams providing care for patients with cardiovascular health needs in a wide variety of healthcare environments. Heart surgery began in 1944 with the first palliative procedure for "blue" babies. The first open heart surgery was performed in 1955 to repair a congenital defect. In the 1950s nurses helped develop specialized operating rooms for heart and lung surgery and cardiac catheterization laboratories. In 1957, one of the world's first coronary care units (CCUs) opened in America. At that time the units were called "heart rooms" or constant care units because nurses provided care around the clock for these vulnerable patients. Both surgical and post-myocardial infarction patients were treated in this environment. Coronary care units provided a model for specialized care where nurses learned about arrhythmia recognition and early defibrillation. Infants and children were typically isolated in specialized areas of pediatric wards, whose nursing staff acquired high levels of skill in yet another important area of cardiovascular health care. As the science of cardiovascular nursing emerged, expectations of care rose among the public, patients, and the healthcare professions.

Today, the field of cardiovascular nursing is exciting and rich with opportunities for nurses to affect the lives of countless patients and families. Nursing practice encompasses the vast needs of patients across the lifespan, from newborns and children to the elderly. Given

The content in this appendix is not current and is of historical significance only.

the prevalence of people who are living with preventable cardio-vascular conditions that are now chronic and debilitating, cardiovas-cular nurses are in a unique position to create prevention programs for individuals and communities. Preventing cardiovascular disease starts in infancy. Helping people avoid obesity, stop smoking, be more active, and eat healthier can significantly reduce morbidity and mor-tality associated with cardiovascular disease. Cardiovascular nurses can and do lead many of these prevention efforts.

Excellence in cardiovascular nursing requires advanced cardiovascu-lar knowledge and skills. This document describes this knowledge base, and thereby provides a framework for developing educational curricula and establishes standards of practice for cardiovascular nurses.

The content in this appendix is not current and is of historical significance only.

CARDIOVASCULAR NURSING SCOPE OF PRACTICE

Definition of Cardiovascular Nursing

Cardiovascular (CV) nursing is specialized nursing care focused on the optimization of cardiovascular health across the lifespan. This care includes prevention, detection, and treatment of cardiovascular disease in individuals, families, communities, and populations of all ages. Cardiovascular health is reflected in a lifestyle or environment that prevents or delays the development or progression of cardiovascular disease.

Cardiovascular nurses are registered nurses who emphasize health promotion, disease and injury prevention, symptom recognition, disease management, and self-care knowledge and adherence in order to improve patient outcomes. Cardiovascular nursing uses evidence-based practice to improve patient functional capacity and quality of life, and to enhance the heart health of communities. Cardiovascular nurses develop, implement, and participate in nursing and multidisciplinary cardiovascular research to advance the prevention, diagnosis, and treatment of cardiovascular disease. Practice-based research by cardiovascular nurses provides a better understanding of the impact of healthcare practices and nursing interventions on patient outcomes.

Key elements of cardiovascular nursing care include the development of programs that promote heart health: the education and counseling of individuals, families, and communities about heart health; interventions, such as exercise, that maintain or improve physiologic, psychological, and psychosocial homeostasis; interventions that facilitate and optimize behavioral change and treatment adherence over time; and advocacy to support patients and families during the planning, implementation, and evaluation of their care.

Cardiovascular nurses also focus on optimizing the manner in which health care is delivered in order to provide exceptional cardiovascular care. Cardiovascular care at the healthcare delivery level emphasizes quality monitoring, collaborative practices, disease management, education, research, and administration. Key elements of cardiovascular nursing care at this level include the development, initiation, and maintenance of systems and processes that promote teamwork, collaboration, efficiency, and patient satisfaction.

The content in this appendix is not current and is of historical significance only.

Cardiovascular nursing research is a well-developed aspect of the cardiovascular nursing role. After years of research by nurses into the varied dimensions of practice described above as well as emerging areas like genomics, cardiovascular nursing research has broadened the scientific foundation of cardiovascular practice and provided evidence of effective approaches to cardiovascular nursing care.

The Evolution of Cardiovascular Nursing Practice

The first scope and standards for cardiovascular nursing were developed and published in 1975 in collaboration with the American Heart Association (AHA), and updated in 1981. Since that time the scope of practice of cardiovascular nursing has expanded dramatically, coinciding with the explosion of new evidence about cardiovascular disease epidemiology and pathophysiology across the lifespan, its assessment, diagnosis, treatment, and outcomes. (These predecessor publications are reproduced in Appendixes B, C, and D.)

The scope of practice initially included hospital-based care for individuals experiencing acute, chronic, and critical cardiovascular illnesses. It has since evolved to include prevention, risk modification, and care across the full spectrum of healthcare settings for those who are stable, those with medically unstable chronic cardiovascular illness, and those with major co-morbidities that affect cardiovascular illness assessment, diagnosis, treatment, and outcomes. The current practice of cardiovascular nursing requires extensive clinical knowledge and expertise to provide highly specialized acute, critical, or end-of-life care to hospitalized patients. The practice has also expanded to include an increased emphasis on prevention of cardiovascular disease, providing interventions and care in diverse settings including ambulatory and home-based venues. Cardiovascular nurses partner with patients, families, and other healthcare providers to enhance self-care utilizing innovative models of symptom and disease management in order to improve patient outcomes.

The greater complexity of cardiovascular disease creates crucial roles for cardiovascular nurses as caregivers, coordinators, educators, administrators, case managers, and quality specialists who optimize patient outcomes associated with specific cardiovascular diagnoses. Cardiovascular nurses provide multiple and complex treatments, many of which are initiated or led by nurses. For example, patient education and counseling may involve knowledge and skills in several cardiovascular subspecialities because many patients have numerous concurrent conditions such as hypertension, coronary artery disease, atrial fibrillation, and systolic heart failure. Thus, education must meet the self-care needs of patients with multiple medical conditions. The cardiovascular nurse must be sufficiently knowledgeable to teach patients and families about multiple topics such as diet, exercise or activity, medications, signs and symptoms of worsening condition, self-management behaviors when signs or symptoms emerge or worsen, when to notify a healthcare provider, the type of healthcare provider to call first, as well as medical and nursing research results, diagnostic testing, and new treatments.

Thus, a cardiovascular nurse seeks to go beyond a general nursing role of one who happens to be caring for patients with cardiovascular illnesses or working in a setting—in any capacity—focused on cardiovascular prevention. Rather, a cardiovascular nurse demonstrates a strong interest in the population, a quest for knowledge, and a desire to increase personal competence in the field. The term *cardiovascular nurse* connotes the expectation of a level of cardiovascular care knowledge (basic or advanced) and skills related to the care setting, that entails synthesis of incoming data, delivery of actions, and evaluation steps that ultimately help individuals or groups attain, maintain, or restore cardiovascular health, or meet a peaceful death.

Cardiovascular nurse roles include increasing levels of responsibility, including the development of advanced practice nursing roles such as clinical nurse specialists (CNSs) and nurse practitioners (NPs). More than a dozen professional organizations serve the educational and professional needs of cardiovascular nurses. This revised scope and standards for cardiovascular nursing document is unique in that it is a unifying effort to describe cardiovascular nursing practice based on the participation and contribution of 14 nursing organizations whose constituency includes cardiovascular nurses. (Summary descriptions and the websites of these organizations are in Appendix A.) This document will serve as a new foundation for cardiovascular nursing that will require ongoing assessment and evaluation, so that it consistently represents the state of the art for cardiovascular nursing practice.

Practice Characteristics

Cardiovascular care is collaborative in nature. Cardiovascular nurses partner with physicians and many other members of the healthcare

The content in this appendix is not current and is of historical significance only.

team in a wide range of practice settings, including acute care, skilled nursing facilities, and home settings. An essential nursing role in these settings is direct or indirect contact with individuals with actual or potential cardiovascular disease. Cardiovascular nurses work at the bedside in acute care settings (emergency, perioperative, acute, progressive, and intensive care settings for children and adults), in transplant programs, in cardiac rehabilitation, in offices and clinics where cardiology or cardiovascular surgery is emphasized, and in community health, home care, and hospice or palliative care. Many cardiovascular nurses work in general practice settings such as family practice, pediatrics, obstetrics, internal medicine, and gerontology practices with large patient populations who are aging and at risk for or who have cardiovascular disease. Cardiovascular nurses work in other diverse settings such as telemonitoring, information technology, cardiac catheterization and electrophysiology laboratories, noninvasive imaging, radiology, exercise testing, heart failure clinics and transplantation programs, and the pharmaceutical and device industries.

Cardiovascular nurses also provide even more specialized cardiovascular care by managing and directing clinics focused on risk reduction, anticoagulation, lipid, hypertension, heart failure, cardiac rhythm management, life-sustaining and lifesaving devices, infusion therapies, genetics, peripartum care, and pediatric or adult congenital heart disease. Because nursing practice may be dictated by the patient population (e.g., pediatric, elderly, hypertension, heart failure) or setting (e.g., critical or ambulatory care), cardiovascular nurse training, professional development, and advanced specialized clinical knowledge and skills must be commensurate with the nursing practice needs of the patient population and setting.

Educational Requirements for General Cardiovascular Nurses

Cardiovascular nurses include licensed registered nurses and advanced practice nurses (nurse practitioners or clinical nurse specialists), nurse educators, administrators, case managers, quality specialists, and researchers. An RN, regardless of specialty, is licensed and authorized by a state, commonwealth, or territory to practice nursing. The RN is educationally prepared for competent practice at the beginning novice level upon graduating from an approved school of nursing and qualified national examination for RN licensure. Since 1965, the American Nurses

The content in this appendix is not current and is of historical significance only.

Association (ANA) has consistently affirmed the baccalaureate degree in nursing as the preferred educational preparation for entry into nursing practice. However, new nurses may enter the profession with diploma, associate, baccalaureate, generic master's, or doctoral degrees.

All RNs begin their education in the science and art of nursing with an overall goal of helping individuals or groups attain, maintain, and restore health whenever possible. Experienced nurses become proficient in one or more practice areas or roles, and may focus on patient care in clinical nursing practice specialties, such as cardiovascular nursing. Specialized cardiovascular knowledge and experience may be acknowledged through an identified certification process, in which specific nursing educational requirements and demonstration of knowledge in cardiovascular nursing practice have been delineated and validated (e.g., the ANCC and ACCN Cardiac/Vascular Nursing exams, or the CCRN Critical Care exam).

Registered nurses may elect to pursue studies for advanced cardiovascular nursing specialization. Educational requirements vary by specialty, role, and educational institution. Upon graduation, cardiovascular nurses may pursue national certification in a variety of direct and indirect care roles (e.g., adult health, critical care, community health, clinical nurse specialist, or nurse practitioner). In response to changing healthcare, education, and regulatory environments, models of education continue to evolve. Advanced practice certification examinations for cardiovascular nursing are currently being developed.

To provide general cardiovascular nursing care, nurses need a broad knowledge base in anatomy, physiology, pharmacology, pharmacogenomics, pharmacotherapeutics, nutrition, psychology, sociology, and developmental theory. The professional cardiovascular general practice nurse requires a specialty knowledge base, as indicated above. Clinical competencies beyond that obtained in basic nursing education include assessment and management of cardiovascular conditions, education and counseling skills for comprehensive cardiovascular risk factor reduction, disease management, and encouraging patients in a lifelong pattern of healthy living.

Competencies in addressing the physiological, psychosocial, educational, and spiritual needs of patients living with chronic cardiovascular illness are essential, including skill in helping patients and families deal with aging and end-of-life issues. Cardiovascular nurses must be

The content in this appendix is not current and is of historical significance only.

knowledgeable of the principles of ethical practice and have resources available to evaluate the merits, risks, and social concerns of cardiovascular interventions. In addition, as part of autonomous cardiovascular nursing practice, nurses must be educated in patient advocacy across the age spectrum. Starting with nutritional support and avoidance of teratogens at conception, education on healthy nutrition and exercise is essential, along with garnering greater public support for the elderly because of their increased incidence of cardiovascular disease.

The core of cardiovascular nursing practice centers on the use of clinical judgment and decision-making based on scientific information and theory, and evidenced-based guidelines as they relate to cardiovascular care. In providing comprehensive care across the continuum from prevention to end of life, the general cardiovascular nurse uses the nursing process to assess individual and group needs, to form an appropriate nursing diagnosis, to design a mutually agreed upon plan of care, to coordinate and provide therapeutic interventions, to document the care, and to evaluate this action plan using a multidisciplinary case management approach.

Strong assessment skills are the foundation of cardiovascular nursing practice. These include both cardiac and vascular system assessment in addition to all affected systems. Intensive knowledge of cardiovascular physiology is necessary, including the principles of electrophysiology and dysrhythmia recognition, as these are required by all cardiovascular nurses to accurately assess and respond appropriately to life-threatening conditions.

With the explosion of knowledge has come complex equipment to evaluate, monitor, and treat cardiovascular patients. This equipment varies in complexity from simple diagnostic tools such as the stethoscope and sphygmomanometer, to complex imaging systems that can diagnose a congenital heart defect before 20 weeks gestational age, reconstruct damaged or defective hearts, and guide catheters into coronary arteries. Patient monitoring systems likewise have evolved from simple bedside monitors of electrocardiograms to implantable devices to document arrhythmias. With the development of small chip microprocessors, cardiac rhythm management devices have become extremely complex and can monitor hemodynamic changes, analyze cardiac rhythms, and provide therapy for potentially fatal arrhythmias. Mechanical circulatory support has evolved from bridge devices for cardiac transplantation to end-stage heart failure treatment for select patient

The content in this appendix is not current and is of historical significance only.

populations. As a result, cardiovascular nurses require a general working knowledge of these aspects of care.

Many general cardiovascular nurses learn to use and monitor the data from catheters and devices associated with medical, surgical, and preventive care for all ages of people with cardiovascular conditions. Examples include pulmonary artery catheters, thoracic impedance or hemodynamic monitoring devices (internal or external systems), cardiac rhythm management devices, and mechanical circulatory support devices. With their expertise in these advanced technologies, cardiovascular nurses can assure patient safety during their use, monitor the function of and manage information provided by the equipment, assess patient responses, and teach patients and families about the temporary and long-term use of these devices.

A strong cardiovascular knowledge base is necessary for cardiovascular administrators, researchers, case managers, transplant coordinators, quality specialists, and educators in cardiovascular disease; they need a thorough preparation in their area of service in addition to nurse provider knowledge.

Advanced Practice Cardiovascular Nursing

Registered nurses with graduate education and advanced specialized clinical knowledge and skills are advanced practice registered nurses (APRNs), including clinical nurse specialists (CNSs) and nurse practitioners (NPs). APRNs have earned an advanced nursing degree and demonstrate a greater depth and breadth of nursing knowledge, synthesis of data, advanced nursing skills, and significant autonomy. Although the scope of practice for RNs and APRNs is distinctly different, there is an overlap in some cardiovascular knowledge and skills.

NPs specializing in cardiovascular care are registered nurses with a master's or doctoral degree as an nurse practitioner. The role requires expanded knowledge and skills for providing expert care to individuals, groups, or populations at risk for or diagnosed with cardiovascular disease. They conduct comprehensive assessments and promote health and prevention of cardiovascular injury and disease. A cardiovascular NP develops differential diagnoses, orders tests and procedures, performs physical examinations, interprets diagnostic and laboratory tests, makes a diagnosis, and prescribes pharmacologic and non-pharmacologic

The content in this appendix is not current and is of historical significance only.

therapies for the direct management and treatment of acute and chronic cardiovascular illness and disease.

Cardiovascular NPs provide evidenced-based health and medical care in primary, acute, and long-term settings, and practice both autonomously and in collaboration with other healthcare professionals to treat and manage cardiovascular health problems. They promote cardiovascular health and disease prevention through patient and community education, advocating for heart-healthy life styles, performing cardiovascular risk assessment, and implementing risk factor modifications. Cardiovascular NPs serve in a variety of settings as researchers, consultants, and patient advocates to individuals, families, groups, and communities.

Cardiovascular CNSs are registered nurses who have graduate-level nursing preparation at the master's or doctoral degree level as a CNS. They are clinical experts in evidence-based cardiovascular nursing practice, treating and managing the health problems of cardiovascular patients and populations. Cardiovascular CNSs practice autonomously, integrating knowledge of disease and medical conditions into the assessment, diagnosis, and treatment of patients' cardiovascular illnesses. They also work collaboratively with other members of the healthcare team.

These nurses design, implement, and evaluate both patient-specific and population-based programs of care. Cardiovascular CNSs provide leadership in advancing the practice of cardiovascular nursing to achieve quality and cost-effective patient outcomes. They lead multidisciplinary groups in designing and implementing innovative alternative solutions that address systems and patient care issues. As direct care providers, cardiovascular CNSs perform comprehensive health assessments, develop differential diagnoses, and may have prescriptive authority, which allows them to prescribe pharmacologic and non-pharmacologic agents for the direct management and treatment of acute and chronic cardiovascular illness and disease. Cardiovascular CNSs serve as patient advocates and educators. They provide expert consultation and education to healthcare providers, and conduct and interpret research to improve practices and enhance patient outcomes.

Continuing Professional Development and Lifelong Learning

Cardiovascular nursing professional development is a lifelong process of active participation by the cardiovascular generalist or advanced

The content in this appendix is not current and is of historical significance only.

practice registered nurse (APRN) in learning to acquire and maintain competence, enhance professional practice, and achieve career goals. Cardiovascular nursing professional development begins with the basic academic nursing preparation and continues throughout the professional life of the cardiovascular nurse.

Lifelong learning, which is the obligation and responsibility of all nurses, is expected and necessary to maintain and increase competency in cardiovascular nursing practice. Continuing competence is essential to the provision of safe, quality health care to cardiovascular patients and ensures that the nurse can perform in a changing healthcare environment. Continuing competence is the hallmark of professionalism and a means by which a professional is held accountable to society. Competence is reflected in the nurse's ability to use their knowledge, skill, judgment, abilities, values, and beliefs to deliver quality care to cardiovascular patients in a variety of situations and practice settings. All cardiovascular patients are entitled to receive care from cardiovascular nurses who maintain professional nursing competence.

Cardiovascular nursing professional development encompasses the domains of academic education, continuing education, and staff development. Academic education consists of courses taken for credit in an institution of higher education that may or may not lead to a degree, completion of a certification program, or individual coursework taken to update oneself in the cardiovascular specialty. Continuing education comprises a systematic professional learning experience designed to augment the knowledge, skills, and abilities, thereby enriching the nurse's contribution to quality health care. Continuing education can be part of a formal academic program, part of staff development, or studying for the purpose of enhancing cardiovascular nursing practice. Staff development is the systematic process of assessment, planning, education, and evaluation that enhances the performance or professional growth of the nurse. Staff development can include continuing education and academic education.

Specialty Certification

Certification in the United States is a voluntary process whereby a nongovernmental agency, such as the American Nurses Credentialing Center (ANCC), the American Association of Critical-Care Nurses Credentialing Center, or another professional organization, recognizes

The content in this appendix is not current and is of historical significance only.

and validates an individual's knowledge, skills, and abilities in a defined area of nursing practice. This professional certification represents the recognition of the excellence and continued competency of the nurse and serves to assure the public of competent professional practice. Certification is accomplished by meeting pre-established standards, usually including the successful completion of an examination.

Nurses who achieve certification in cardiovascular nursing assure clients, patients, and families that they possess the knowledge and skills needed to give excellent cardiovascular care. Cardiovascular nursing examinations incorporate the domains of practice described above. Some cardiovascular nurses may choose to attain interdisciplinary certifications which demonstrate expertise in use of specific technologies (e.g., interrogation and reprogramming of permanent pacemakers) or skills (e.g., clinical management of organ transplant recipients, healthcare quality management). Advanced practice certification examinations for cardiovascular nursing are not available at this time, but are currently being developed.

Future Considerations

A host of issues and trends in health care influence specialty nursing care for individuals and families at risk for or with cardiovascular health problems. As the baby boomers age, the sheer volume of people requiring cardiovascular care will have a significant impact on healthcare resources and demands for services through 2020, and will directly affect the cardiovascular nursing profession. New discoveries about the genetic and pathophysiologic origins of disease and how they interact with environment and lifestyle have added to our already vast knowledge, challenging those in the nursing profession to stay well-informed for their roles in providing care, advocating for patient needs, and teaching patients and their families. Emerging science about novel risk factors that increase the probability of cardiovascular disease, new diagnostic tests and treatments, and advances in genomics and genetics, including pharmacogenomics, will shape treatment choices in the future. Cardiovascular nurses are challenged to engage in lifelong learning in order to keep abreast of the rapidly developing science and to always provide evidence-based nursing care. The translation of new knowledge and evidence must be accelerated.

The content in this appendix is not current and is of historical significance only.

The explosion of new information has heightened the importance of the use of evidence in providing care and counseling for patients about their therapeutic options. Thus, maintaining current knowledge in this era of evidence-based practice is both challenging and essential. A variety of issues related to the current nursing workforce and work environments warrant attention in planning for future cardiovascular health care. The continuing shortage of nurses, aggravated by the aging nursing workforce, is well-documented. Work environments for nurses must be transformed in order to retain experienced practitioners. Nurses must be involved in decisions related to creating patient care systems and healthy work environments. Continued efforts and funding to support nursing education are also essential to ensure adequate numbers of knowledgeable and competent cardiovascular nurses. New specialized healthcare provider roles increase the risk of fragmented, discontinuous care and poor communication. Enhanced skills in interdisciplinary communication and collaboration will be required of nurses in order to ensure patient safety and coordination of care.

Projected shortages of primary care physicians and changes in medical education provide opportunities for advanced practice nurses but deplete the number of nurses available at the bedside. At the same time, physician shortages provide an opportunity for advanced practice nurses to collaborate with physicians, registered nurses, and healthcare executives to reconfigure care systems and develop structures and processes that promote evidence-based practice. Advanced practice nurses are also integral to efforts to improve interdisciplinary communication, interpret and accelerate the application of evidence to patient care, conduct research, and improve outcomes of care.

Issues specific to care environments include technology, work force, safety, and patient transitions. As the rate of technological advances increases, cardiovascular nurses need to be competent in the application and evaluation of technology, which incorporates ethical decisions in the use of the technology. The incidence of adverse events and medical errors in all healthcare settings mandates a continued emphasis on safety and quality initiatives in caring for patients with cardiovascular healthcare needs.

Fragmentation of care contributes to a greater need for nurses to be able to provide seamless care and excellent communication as patients move between acute care and community or home settings. The shift

The content in this appendix is not current and is of historical significance only.

of hospital-based therapies to ambulatory and home care settings requires a competent and knowledgeable nursing workforce, regardless of the setting where patients receive care. Telehealth technologies, which help nurses to assess, monitor, and treat patients remotely, require technological expertise, knowledge of transitional care issues, and vigilance to ensure continuing communication with patients and families about their nursing care needs.

The growing number of infants and elderly patients with complex cardiovascular disease complicated by comorbidities, combined with shortened hospital stays, will require cardiovascular nurses to address the complexities involved in the transition of patients from hospital to home or long-term care or its future alternatives. Increased communication between ambulatory and home-based care providers, improved discharge planning, and better training of families and caregivers to manage illness and appropriately access the healthcare system are needed.

The complexity of the healthcare system remains a challenge for many patients and families who desire a more active role in decision-making about health. Self-care and increased healthcare consumerism provide nurses with unique opportunities to influence outcomes. Quality of life, and how it affects patients' decisions about new therapies, is an important consideration, as are the knowledge, skills, and emotions of the family or caregiver. Advances in science, and patient longevity, afford nurses even greater opportunity to influence target audiences at multiple points across the life span. Emphasis on the patient's personal responsibility for improving health can foster stronger partnerships with healthcare decision-makers considering various treatment options.

Initiatives in health promotion and disease prevention continue to be under-funded by insurance companies in most healthcare systems. The need to justify costly health care with improved outcomes has renewed the focus on prevention. However, standardized coding systems downplay interdisciplinary efforts, resulting in decreased reimbursement for such efforts and limiting innovation to meet these goals. Increasing financial burdens on consumers, employers, and government resources are providing opportunities for nurses to become part of future solutions. Given the prevalence of people who are living with chronic, preventable cardiovascular conditions, cardiovascular nurses are in a unique position to create programs for individuals and communities.

The content in this appendix is not current and is of historical significance only.

Preventing cardiovascular disease starts in infancy. Helping people avoid obesity, stop smoking, be more active, and eat better can significantly reduce morbidity and mortality associated with cardiovascular disease. Cardiovascular nurses will need to apply emerging knowledge of how successful behavioral change happens if they are to lead patients to adopt healthier lifestyles.

The healthcare needs of underserved and ethnically diverse populations provide both opportunities and responsibilities for nurses. Advanced practice nurses with expertise in physiology, medicine, and behavioral change contribute to improvements in the health of patients and families. Cardiovascular nurses bring unique knowledge, skills, and expertise that can be used to create innovative programs for improving the health of patients, families, and communities. Together, this competent and caring nursing workforce has the knowledge and expertise needed to care for the nearly 80 million people who are living with cardiovascular disease in the United States.

This current scope and standards for cardiovascular nursing will of necessity be a living document, continually updated as our understanding and management of cardiovascular disease advances. In its current form it should provide the foundation for sound cardiovascular nursing practice.

Additional Content

For a better appreciation of the historical and professional context underlying the publication of *Cardiovascular Nursing: Scope and Standards of Practice*, the contents of three predecessor publications—the successive 1975 and 1981 editions of the standards of cardiovascular nursing practice, along with the related 1993 scope of cardiac rehabilitation practice—have been included in the text and indexed with the current content of this edition.

- Appendix B: *The Scope of Cardiac Rehabilitation Practice* (1993)
- Appendix C: *Standards of Cardiovascular Nursing Practice* (1981)
- Appendix D: *Standards of Cardiovascular Nursing Practice* (1975)

Standards of Cardiovascular Nursing Practice

Standards of Practice

Standard 1. Assessment
The cardiovascular registered nurse collects comprehensive data pertinent to the patient's health or the situation.

Measurement Criteria:

The cardiovascular registered nurse:

- Collects data in a systematic and ongoing process.

- Involves the patient, family, other healthcare providers, and environment as appropriate in holistic data collection.

- Is involved in assessment of patients of all ages across the continuum of care from acute to community care.

- Prioritizes data collection activities based on the patient's immediate condition, or anticipated needs of the patient or situation.

- Uses developmentally appropriate evidence-based assessment techniques and instruments in collecting pertinent data.

- Uses analytical models and problem-solving tools.

- Synthesizes available data, information, and knowledge relevant to the situation to identify patterns and variances.

- Documents relevant data in a retrievable format.

Additional Measurement Criteria for the Advanced Practice Registered Nurse:

The advanced practice cardiovascular registered nurse:

- Initiates and interprets diagnostic tests and procedures relevant to the patient's current status.

The content in this appendix is not current and is of historical significance only.

STANDARD 2. DIAGNOSIS
The cardiovascular registered nurse analyzes the assessment data to determine the nursing diagnoses or health-related issues.

Measurement Criteria:

The cardiovascular registered nurse:

- Derives the diagnoses or issues based on assessment data that reflect the patient's current clinical condition.

- Systematically compares and contrasts clinical findings with normal and abnormal variations.

- Derives diagnoses encompassing:

  - The patient's identified or potential physiological, psychological, and developmental problems.

  - The needs of the child or adolescent to attend school.

  - The needs of the elderly patient regarding integration into post-hospital or long-term care.

  - The support and educational needs of the family or designated care provider.

  - Any present or potential environmental problems.

- Refines and revises diagnoses regularly, based on data subsequently collected.

- Discusses diagnoses and cardiovascular risk factors with the patient, family, caregivers, members of the interdisciplinary team, and other healthcare providers when possible and appropriate.

- Documents diagnoses or issues in a manner that facilitates the determination of the expected outcomes and plan.

Additional Measurement Criteria for the Advanced Practice Registered Nurse:

The advanced practice cardiovascular registered nurse:

- Systematically compares and contrasts clinical findings with normal and abnormal variations and developmental events in formulating a differential diagnosis.

- Utilizes complex data and information obtained during interview, examination, and diagnostic procedures in identifying diagnoses.

- Assists staff in developing and maintaining competency in the diagnostic process.

The content in this appendix is not current and is of historical significance only.

STANDARD 3. OUTCOMES IDENTIFICATION

The cardiovascular registered nurse identifies expected outcomes for a plan individualized to the patient or the situation.

Measurement Criteria:

The cardiovascular registered nurse:

- Identifies expected outcomes mutually with the patient, family, and other healthcare providers. Expected outcomes are patient-oriented, developmentally appropriate, evidenced-based, and attainable given the patient's and family's present and potential capabilities.

- Derives culturally and age-appropriate expected outcomes from the diagnoses.

- Considers associated risks, benefits, costs, current scientific evidence, and clinical expertise when formulating expected outcomes.

- Defines expected outcomes in terms of the patient, patient values, ethical considerations, environment, or situation with such consideration as associated risks, benefits and costs, and current scientific evidence.

- Includes a time estimate for attainment of expected outcomes.

- Develops expected outcomes that provide direction for continuity of care.

- Modifies expected outcomes based on changes in the status of the patient or evaluation of the situation.

- Documents expected outcomes as measurable goals.

- Implements national consensus-based clinical guidelines.

Additional Measurement Criteria for the Advanced Practice Registered Nurse:

The advanced practice cardiovascular registered nurse:

- Identifies expected outcomes that incorporate scientific evidence and are achievable through implementation of evidence-based practices.

- Identifies expected outcomes that incorporate cost and clinical effectiveness, patient satisfaction, and continuity and consistency among providers.

- Supports the use of clinical guidelines linked to positive patient outcomes.

STANDARD 4. PLANNING
The cardiovascular registered nurse develops a plan that prescribes strategies and alternatives to attain expected outcomes.

Measurement Criteria:

The cardiovascular registered nurse:

- Develops an individualized cardiovascular plan considering patient characteristics, developmental level, and situation (e.g., age- and culturally appropriate, environmentally sensitive).

- Participates in the design and development of multidisciplinary and interdisciplinary processes to address the situation or issue.

- Contributes to the development and continuous improvement of organizational systems that support the planning process.

- Supports the integration of clinical, human, and financial resources to enhance and complete the decision-making processes.

- Develops the plan in conjunction with the patient, family, and others, synthesizing patients' values and beliefs, developmental level, and coping style.

- Includes strategies in the plan that address each of the identified diagnoses or issues, which may include strategies for promotion and restoration of health and prevention of illness, injury, and disease.

- Provides for continuity in the plan.

- Incorporates an implementation pathway or timeline in the plan.

- Establishes the plan priorities with the patient, family, and others as appropriate.

- Utilizes the plan to provide direction to other members of the healthcare team.

- Defines the plan to reflect current statutes, rules and regulations, and standards of cardiovascular nursing practice.

- Integrates current trends and research affecting care in the planning process.

- Considers the economic impact of the plan for the patient, family, caregivers, or other affected parties.

- Uses standardized language or recognized terminology to document the plan.

The content in this appendix is not current and is of historical significance only.

Additional Measurement Criteria for the Advanced Practice Registered Nurse:

The advanced practice cardiovascular registered nurse:

- Identifies assessment, diagnostic strategies, and therapeutic interventions in the plan that reflect current evidence, including data, research, literature, and expert clinical knowledge.

- Selects or designs strategies to meet the multifaceted needs of complex patients.

- Includes the synthesis of patients' values and beliefs regarding nursing and medical therapies in the plan.

The content in this appendix is not current and is of historical significance only.

STANDARD 5. IMPLEMENTATION
The cardiovascular registered nurse implements the identified plan.

Measurement Criteria:

The cardiovascular registered nurse:

- Implements the plan in a safe and timely manner.

- Implements the plan using principles and concepts of project or systems management.

- Fosters organizational systems that support implementation of the plan.

- Documents implementation and any modifications, including changes or omissions, of the identified plan.

- Utilizes evidence-based interventions and treatments specific to the diagnosis or problem.

- Facilitates utilization of systems and community resources to implement the plan.

- Collaborates with nursing colleagues and other disciplines to implement the plan.

- Incorporates new knowledge and strategies to initiate change in nursing care practices if desired outcomes are not achieved.

Additional Measurement Criteria for the Advanced Practice Registered Nurse:

The advanced practice cardiovascular registered nurse:

- Facilitates utilization of systems and community resources to implement the plan.

- Supports collaboration with nursing colleagues and other disciplines to implement the plan.

- Incorporates new knowledge and strategies to initiate change in nursing care practices if desired outcomes are not achieved.

STANDARD 5A. COORDINATION OF CARE
The cardiovascular registered nurse coordinates care delivery.

Measurement Criteria:

The cardiovascular registered nurse:

- Provides leadership in the coordination of multidisciplinary health care for integrated delivery of patient care services.

- Documents the coordination of care.

- Synthesizes data and information to facilitate necessary system and community support measures, including environmental modifications.

- Coordinates system and community resources that enhance delivery of care across the continuum.

Measurement Criteria for the Advanced Practice Registered Nurse:

The advanced practice cardiovascular registered nurse:

- Provides leadership in the coordination of multidisciplinary health care for integrated delivery of patient care services.

- Synthesizes data and information to prescribe necessary system and community support measures, including environmental modifications.

- Coordinates system and community resources that enhance delivery of care across continuums.

The content in this appendix is not current and is of historical significance only.

STANDARD 5B. HEALTH TEACHING AND HEALTH PROMOTION
The cardiovascular registered nurse employs strategies to promote health and a safe environment.

Measurement Criteria:

The cardiovascular registered nurse:

- Provides health teaching that addresses such topics as healthy lifestyles, risk-reducing behaviors, developmental needs, activities of daily living, and preventive self-care.

- Uses health promotion and health teaching methods appropriate to the situation and the patient's developmental level, learning needs, readiness, ability to learn, literacy level, language preference, and culture.

- Seeks opportunities for feedback and evaluation of the effectiveness of the strategies used.

Additional Measurement Criteria for the Advanced Practice Registered Nurse:

The advanced practice cardiovascular registered nurse:

- Synthesizes empirical evidence on risk behaviors, learning theories, behavioral change theories, motivational theories, epidemiology, and other related theories and frameworks when designing health information and patient education.

- Designs health information and patient education appropriate to the patient's developmental level, learning needs, readiness to learn, and cultural values and beliefs.

- Evaluates health information resources, such as Internet sites, within the area of practice for accuracy, readability, and comprehensibility to help patients access quality health information.

The content in this appendix is not current and is of historical significance only.

STANDARD 5C. CONSULTATION

The cardiovascular registered nurse provides consultation to influence the identified plan, enhance the abilities of others, and effect change.

Measurement Criteria:

The cardiovascular registered nurse:

- Synthesizes clinical data, theoretical frameworks, and evidence when providing consultation.

- Facilitates the effectiveness of a consultation by involving the patient and family in decision-making and negotiating role responsibilities.

- Communicates consultation recommendations to facilitate change.

- Communicates consultation recommendations that influence the identified plan, facilitates understanding by involved stakeholders, enhances the work of others, and effects change.

Additional Measurement Criteria for the Advanced Practice Registered Nurse:

The advanced practice cardiovascular registered nurse:

- Synthesizes complex clinical data, theoretical frameworks, and evidence when providing consultation.

- Facilitates the effectiveness of a consultation by involving the patient and family in decision-making and negotiating role responsibilities.

- Facilitates the effectiveness of a consultation by conducting research and disseminating research findings to enhance interaction meaningfulness (psychosocial or clinical outcomes).

- Directs consultation recommendations that facilitate change.

The content in this appendix is not current and is of historical significance only.

STANDARD 5D. PRESCRIPTIVE AUTHORITY AND TREATMENT
The advanced practice cardiovascular registered nurse uses prescriptive authority, procedures, referrals, treatments, and therapies in accordance with state and federal laws and regulations.

Measurement Criteria for the Advanced Practice Registered Nurse:

The advanced practice cardiovascular registered nurse:

- Prescribes evidence-based treatments, therapies, and procedures considering the patient's comprehensive healthcare needs.

- Prescribes pharmacologic agents based on a current knowledge of pharmacology and physiology.

- Prescribes specific pharmacological agents or treatments based on clinical indicators, the patient's status and needs, and the results of diagnostic and laboratory tests.

- Evaluates therapeutic and potential adverse effects of pharmacological and non-pharmacological treatments.

- Provides patients with information about intended effects and potential adverse effects of proposed prescriptive therapies.

- Provides information about costs, and alternative treatments and procedures, as appropriate.

The content in this appendix is not current and is of historical significance only.

STANDARD 6. EVALUATION
The cardiovascular registered nurse evaluates progress towards attainment of outcomes.

Measurement Criteria:

The cardiovascular registered nurse:

- Conducts a systematic, ongoing, and criterion-based evaluation of the outcomes in relation to the structures and processes prescribed by the plan and the indicated timeline.

- Includes the patient and others involved in the care or situation in the evaluative process.

- Evaluates the effectiveness of the planned strategies in relation to patient responses and the attainment of the expected outcomes.

- Documents the results of the evaluation.

- Uses ongoing assessment data to revise the diagnoses, the outcomes, the plan, and the implementation as needed.

- Disseminates the results to the patient and others involved in the care or situation, as appropriate, in accordance with state and federal laws and regulations.

Additional Measurement Criteria for the Advanced Practice Registered Nurse:

The advanced practice cardiovascular registered nurse:

- Evaluates the accuracy of the diagnosis and effectiveness of the interventions in relationship to the patient's attainment of expected outcomes.

- Synthesizes the results of the evaluation to determine the impact of the plan on the affected patients, families, groups, communities, and institutions.

- Uses the results of the evaluation to make or recommend process or structural changes including policy, procedure, or protocol documentation, as appropriate.

The content in this appendix is not current and is of historical significance only.

STANDARDS OF PROFESSIONAL PERFORMANCE

STANDARD 7. QUALITY OF PRACTICE
The cardiovascular registered nurse systematically enhances the quality and effectiveness of nursing practice.

Measurement Criteria:

The cardiovascular registered nurse:

- Demonstrates quality by documenting the application of the nursing process in a responsible, accountable, and ethical manner.

- Uses the results of quality improvement activities to initiate changes in nursing practice and in the healthcare delivery system.

- Uses creativity and innovation in nursing practice to improve care delivery.

- Incorporates new knowledge to initiate changes in nursing practice if desired outcomes are not achieved.

- Obtains and maintains professional certification if available in the area of expertise.

- Designs and participates in quality improvement activities. Such activities may include:

  - Identifying aspects of practice important for quality monitoring.

  - Using indicators developed to monitor quality and effectiveness of nursing practice.

  - Collecting data to monitor quality and effectiveness of nursing practice.

  - Analyzing quality data to identify opportunities for improving nursing practice.

  - Formulating recommendations to improve nursing practice or outcomes.

  - Implementing activities to enhance the quality of nursing practice.

Continued ▶

The content in this appendix is not current and is of historical significance only.

- Developing, implementing, and evaluating policies, procedures, and guidelines to improve the quality of practice.

- Participating on interdisciplinary teams to evaluate clinical care or health services.

- Participating in efforts to minimize costs and unnecessary duplication.

- Analyzing factors related to safety, satisfaction, effectiveness, and cost–benefit options.

- Analyzing organizational systems for barriers.

- Implementing processes to remove or decrease barriers within organizational systems.

Additional Measurement Criteria for the Advanced Practice Registered Nurse:

The advanced practice cardiovascular registered nurse:

- Obtains and maintains professional certification if available in the area of expertise.

- Designs quality improvement initiatives.

- Implements initiatives to evaluate the need for change.

- Evaluates the practice environment and quality of nursing care in relation to existing evidence, identifying opportunities for the generation and use of research.

The content in this appendix is not current and is of historical significance only.

STANDARD 8. EDUCATION
The cardiovascular registered nurse attains knowledge and competency that reflects current nursing practice.

Measurement Criteria:

The cardiovascular registered nurse:

- Participates in ongoing educational activities related to appropriate knowledge bases and professional issues.

- Demonstrates a commitment to lifelong learning through self-reflection and inquiry to identify learning needs.

- Seeks experiences that reflect current practice in order to maintain skills and competence in clinical practice or role performance.

- Acquires knowledge and skills appropriate to the specialty area, practice setting, role, or situation.

- Maintains professional records that provide evidence of competency and lifelong learning.

- Seeks experiences and formal and independent learning activities to maintain and develop clinical and professional skills and knowledge.

- Obtains and maintains professional certification if available in the area of expertise.

Additional Measurement Criteria for the Advanced Practice Registered Nurse:

The advanced practice cardiovascular registered nurse:

- Uses current healthcare research findings and other evidence to expand clinical knowledge, enhance role performance, and increase knowledge of professional issues.

The content in this appendix is not current and is of historical significance only.

STANDARD 9. PROFESSIONAL PRACTICE EVALUATION

The cardiovascular registered nurse evaluates one's own nursing practice in relation to professional practice standards and guidelines, relevant statutes, rules, and regulations.

Measurement Criteria:

The cardiovascular registered nurse:

- Applies knowledge of current practice standards, guidelines, statutes, rules, and regulations in practice.

- Provides age- and developmentally appropriate care in a culturally and ethnically sensitive manner.

- Engages in self-evaluation of practice on a regular basis, identifying areas of strength as well as areas in which professional development would be beneficial.

- Obtains informal feedback regarding one's own practice from patients, peers, professional colleagues, and others.

- Participates in systematic peer review as appropriate.

- Takes action to achieve goals identified during the evaluation process.

- Provides rationales for practice beliefs, decisions, and actions as part of the informal and formal evaluation processes.

Additional Measurement Criteria for the Advanced Practice Registered Nurse:

The advanced practice cardiovascular registered nurse:

- Engages in a formal process seeking feedback regarding one's own practice from patients, peers, professional colleagues, and others.

STANDARD 10. COLLEGIALITY

The cardiovascular registered nurse interacts with, and contributes to the professional development of, peers and colleagues.

Measurement Criteria:

The cardiovascular registered nurse:

- Shares knowledge and skills with peers and colleagues as evidenced by such activities as patient care conferences or presentations at formal or informal meetings.

- Mentors other registered nurses and colleagues as appropriate.

- Provides peers with feedback regarding their practice and role performance.

- Interacts with peers and colleagues to enhance one's own professional nursing practice and role performance.

- Actively participates in multidisciplinary teams that contribute to role development and nursing practice.

- Maintains compassionate and caring relationships with peers and colleagues.

- Contributes to an environment that is conducive to the education of healthcare professionals.

- Contributes to a supportive and healthy work environment.

Additional Measurement Criteria for the Advanced Practice Registered Nurse:

The advanced practice cardiovascular registered nurse:

- Models expert practice to multidisciplinary team members and healthcare consumers.

- Mentors other registered nurses and colleagues as appropriate.

- Participates in multidisciplinary teams that contribute to role development and advanced nursing practice and health care.

The content in this appendix is not current and is of historical significance only.

Standard 11. Collaboration
The cardiovascular registered nurse collaborates with the patient, the family, and others in the conduct of nursing practice.

Measurement Criteria:

The cardiovascular registered nurse:

- Communicates with patient, family, and healthcare providers regarding patient care and the nurse's role in the provision of that care.

- Collaborates in creating a documented plan focused on outcomes and decisions related to care and delivery of services that indicates communication with patients, families, and others.

- Consults with other disciplines to enhance patient care through multidisciplinary activities such as education, consultation, management, technological development, or research opportunities.

- Partners with others to effect change and generate positive outcomes through knowledge of the patient or situation.

- Documents referrals, including provisions for continuity of care.

Additional Measurement Criteria for the Advanced Practice Registered Nurse:

The advanced practice cardiovascular registered nurse:

- Partners with other disciplines to enhance patient care through interdisciplinary activities such as education, consultation, management, technological development, or research opportunities.

- Facilitates a multidisciplinary process with other members of the healthcare team.

- Documents plan of care communications, rationales for plan of care changes, and collaborative discussions to improve patient care.

The content in this appendix is not current and is of historical significance only.

Standard 12. Ethics

The cardiovascular registered nurse integrates ethical provisions into all areas of practice.

Measurement Criteria:

The cardiovascular registered nurse:

- Uses *Code of Ethics for Nurses with Interpretive Statements* (ANA 2001) to guide practice.
- Delivers care in a manner that preserves and protects patient autonomy, dignity, and rights.
- Maintains patient confidentiality within legal and regulatory parameters.
- Serves as a patient advocate assisting patients in developing skills for self-advocacy.
- Maintains a therapeutic and professional patient–nurse relationship within appropriate professional role boundaries.
- Demonstrates a commitment to practicing self-care, managing stress, and connecting with self and others.
- Contributes to resolving ethical issues of patients, colleagues, or systems as evidenced in such activities as participating on ethics committees.
- Reports illegal, incompetent, or impaired practices.

Additional Measurement Criteria for the Advanced Practice Registered Nurse:

The advanced practice cardiovascular registered nurse:

- Informs patients of the risks, benefits, and outcomes of healthcare regimens.
- Participates in interdisciplinary teams that address ethical risks, benefits, and outcomes.
- Develops or facilitates nursing research related to ethical issues that emerge during patient care experiences.

The content in this appendix is not current and is of historical significance only.

STANDARD 13. RESEARCH
The cardiovascular registered nurse integrates research findings into practice.

Measurement Criteria:

The cardiovascular registered nurse:

- Utilizes the best available evidence, including research findings, to guide practice decisions.

- Actively participates in research activities at various levels appropriate to the nurse's level of education and position. Such activities may include:

  - Identifying clinical problems specific to nursing research (patient care and nursing practice).

  - Participating in data collection (surveys, pilot projects, and formal studies).

  - Participating in a formal committee or program.

  - Sharing research or findings with peers and others.

  - Conducting research.

  - Critically analyzing and interpreting research for application to practice.

  - Using research findings in the development of policies, procedures, and standards of practice in patient care.

  - Incorporating research as a basis for learning.

Additional Measurement Criteria for the Advanced Practice Registered Nurse:

The advanced practice cardiovascular registered nurse:

- Contributes to nursing knowledge by conducting or synthesizing research that discovers, examines, and evaluates knowledge, theories, criteria, and creative approaches to improve healthcare practice.

- Formally disseminates research findings through activities such as presentations, publications, consultation, and journal clubs.

- Encourages and facilitates nursing research of cardiovascular care topics by mentoring the registered nurse.

The content in this appendix is not current and is of historical significance only.

STANDARD 14. RESOURCE UTILIZATION
The cardiovascular registered nurse considers factors related to safety, effectiveness, cost, and impact on practice in the planning and delivery of nursing services.

Measurement Criteria:

The cardiovascular registered nurse:

- Utilizes organizational and community resources to formulate multidisciplinary or interdisciplinary plans of care.

- Evaluates factors such as safety, effectiveness, availability, cost and benefits, efficiencies, and impact on practice when choosing among practice options that would result in the same expected outcome.

- Assists the patient and family in identifying and securing appropriate and available services to address health-related needs.

- Assigns or delegates tasks, based on the needs and condition of the patient, potential for harm, stability of the patient's condition, complexity of the task, and predictability of the outcome.

- Promotes activities that assist the patient and family in becoming informed consumers about the options, costs, risks, and benefits of treatment and care.

- Develops evaluation strategies to demonstrate cost effectiveness, cost-benefit, and efficiency factors associated with excellence in nursing practice.

Additional Measurement Criteria for the Advanced Practice Registered Nurse:

The advanced practice cardiovascular registered nurse:

- Utilizes organizational and community resources to formulate multidisciplinary or interdisciplinary plans of care.

- Develops innovative solutions for patient care problems that address effective resource utilization and maintenance of quality.

- Develops evaluation strategies to demonstrate cost effectiveness, cost benefit, and efficiency factors associated with nursing practice.

The content in this appendix is not current and is of historical significance only.

STANDARD 15. LEADERSHIP
The cardiovascular registered nurse provides leadership in the professional practice setting and the profession.

Measurement Criteria:

The cardiovascular registered nurse:

- Works to influence decision-making bodies to improve patient care.

- Engages in teamwork as a team player and a team builder.

- Works to create and maintain healthy work environments in local, regional, national, or international communities.

- Displays the ability to define a clear vision, the associated goals, and a plan to implement and measure progress.

- Demonstrates a commitment to continuous, lifelong learning for self and others.

- Teaches others to succeed by mentoring and other strategies.

- Exhibits creativity and flexibility through times of change.

- Demonstrates energy, excitement, and a passion for quality work.

- Willingly accepts mistakes by self and others, thereby creating a culture in which risk-taking is not only safe, but expected.

- Inspires loyalty through valuing of people as the most precious asset in an organization.

- Directs the coordination of care across settings and among care-givers, including oversight of licensed and unlicensed personnel in any assigned or delegated tasks.

- Serves in key roles in the work setting by participating in committees, councils, and administrative teams.

- Promotes advancement of the profession through participation in professional organizations.

The content in this appendix is not current and is of historical significance only.

Additional Measurement Criteria for the Advanced Practice Registered Nurse:

The advanced practice cardiovascular registered nurse:

- Works to influence decision-making bodies to improve patient care.

- Provides direction to enhance the effectiveness of the healthcare team.

- Initiates and revises protocols or guidelines to reflect evidence-based practice, to reflect accepted changes in care management, or to address emerging problems.

- Promotes communication of information and advancement of the profession through writing, publishing, and presentations for professional or lay audiences.

- Designs innovations to effect change in practice and improve health outcomes.

Index

Note: Entries with [2008] indicate an entry from *Cardiovascular Nursing: Scope and Standards of Practice (2008)*, reproduced in Appendix A. That information is not current but included for historical value only.

A

AACN. *See* American Association of Critical-Care Nurses (AACN) Certification Corporation

AAHFN-CB. *See* American Association of Heart Failure Nurses Certification Board (AAHFN-CB)

Abilities in cardiovascular nursing practice, 13, 17, 36, 38, 44, 45, 52, 77, 78, 89, 102
    See also Knowledge, skills, abilities, and judgment

Accountability in cardiovascular nursing practice, 17, 51

Advanced Heart Failure team, 18

Advanced practice registered nurses (APRNs) in cardiovascular nursing practice, 11–12, 75–76
    assessment competencies, 28
        measurement criteria [2008], 82
    collaboration competencies, 53–54
        measurement criteria [2008], 98
    collegiality competencies
        measurement criteria [2008], 97

    consultation competencies, 38
        measurement criteria [2008], 90
    coordination of care competencies, 35
        measurement criteria [2008], 88
    diagnosis competencies, 29
        measurement criteria [2008], 83
    education competencies, 45
        measurement criteria [2008], 95
    environmental health competencies, 58
    ethics competencies, 43
        measurement criteria [2008], 99
    evaluation competencies, 40–41
        measurement criteria [2008], 92
    evidence-based practice and research competencies, 47
    health teaching and health promotion competencies, 36–37
        measurement criteria [2008], 89
    implementation competencies, 34
        measurement criteria [2008], 87
    leadership competencies, 51–52
        measurement criteria [2008], 103
    outcomes identification competencies, 30
        measurement criteria [2008], 84
    planning competencies, 32
        measurement criteria [2008], 86